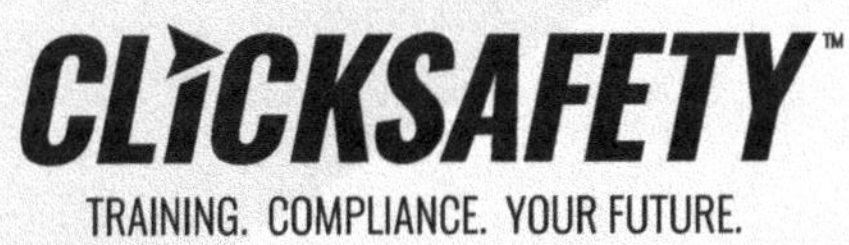

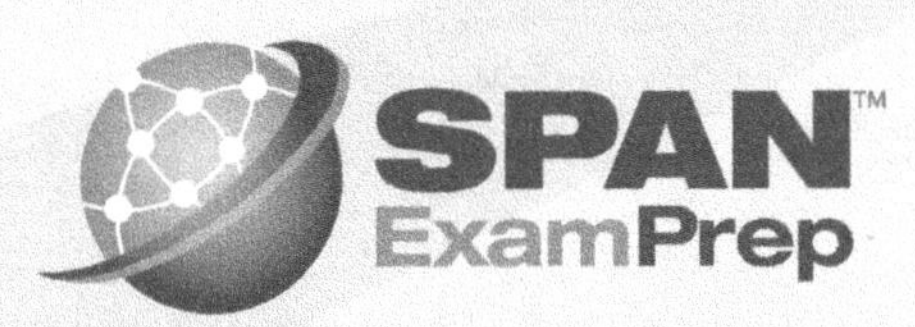

Prep Your Way

Workshops | Online Courses | Workbooks

Associate Safety Professional (ASP)

Certified Instructional Trainer (CIT)

Certified Hazardous Materials Manager (CHMM)

Construction Health and Safety Technician (CHST)

Certified Industrial Hygienist (CIH)

Certified Safety Professional (CSP)

Occupational Hygiene and Safety Technologist (OHST)

Safety Management Specialist (SMS)

Safety Trained Supervisor (STS)

Safety Trained Supervisor Construction (STSC)

SPAN™ Exam Prep is the leading certification exam study solution to prepare safety professionals for exams from the Board of Certified Safety Professionals (BCSP). This BCSP exam prep helps professionals achieve important career goals through advancing competencies for safety management excellence. As the leader in BCSP exam preparation since 1992, SPAN offers live workshops, online courses and workbooks. The self-directed study materials are designed for professionals looking to gain critical knowledge, study techniques, and testing strategies to pass certification examinations.

www.spansafety.com

Dedicated to All Safety, Health and Environmental Professionals

Striving to Protect

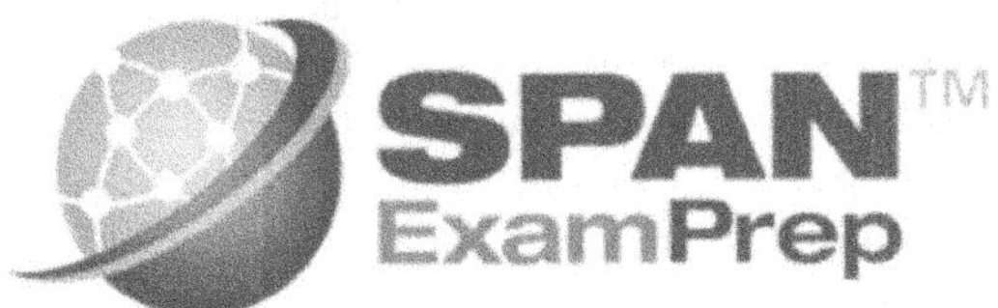

www.spansafety.com

This Publication may not cover every aspect of the certification process and is not intended as a guarantee that the user will pass an exam or become certified.

The information contained in this study workbook is intended to be used in preparation for the Certified Industrial Hygienist® examination and should not be used as an authority in the professional practice of safety, health or environmental compliance.

The Certified Industrial Hygienist® (CIH®) Certification is a registered trademark of the American Board of Industrial Hygienists (ABIH).

The opinions expressed are those of the authors and no guarantee, warranty, or other representation is made as to the absolute correctness or sufficiency of any information contained in this study workbook.

Daniel J. Snyder, Ed.D, CSP, SMS, CHMM, OHST, CET
Tim C. Sterling, MPH, CIH, CSP, OHST

Introduction

There are three major goals of this workbook:

1. Enhance skills, knowledge and abilities as an occupational health and safety professional.
2. Provide preparation for the CIH® examination.
3. Facilitate successful passing of the CIH® examination.

This workbook is designed to be used as a resource for self-directed study in preparation for the CIH exam. In the fast track workshop conducted by SPAN™ International Training, LLC, participants are provided expert guidance and use the same content presented in these workbooks. This curriculum is also used in the online SPAN™ CertBoK® Exam Learning Management System (LMS).

Workshops are conducted periodically throughout the year so professionals can take the examination as soon as they are prepared. Visit the SPAN website for workshop dates and locations: www.spansafety.com.

The workbook is divided into two volumes designed for self-study and facilitated professional development workshops. After each section of the workbook, there are fully developed explanations for the answer selected for each question. In many cases, information about all the selections offered as possible answers will be included to assist in developing a better understanding of the subject. Each section is designed to allow the safety professional to measure progress during the extended program of self-study that is normally required to pass the CIH certification exam.

Considerable effort has been made to fully develop and explain the concepts and techniques discussed. However, given the differences in the background and experience of the safety practitioners sitting for the CIH examination, it is impossible to explain all concepts to all candidates. The materials are based on the exam blueprint and subject matter expertise.

After reviewing the workbook, you should identify your individual knowledge gaps and establish a study plan. There are voluminous resources available for each domain of the exam blueprint. Simply stated, chance favors the prepared mind and candidates should have a study plan. Budget adequate time to master the material.

This workbook is designed to optimize study time. There is no extraneous or "nice to know" information in this workbook. All of the information is important. Concentrating on the areas emphasized in the text should reduce research and study time considerably.

SPAN™ conducts ongoing research and development to ensure the accuracy and quality of the curriculum based on the exam blueprint. ***This workbook does not contain actual CIH test questions.*** The curriculum is designed using a multiple-choice question and answer learning format with detailed explanations that are representative of competencies reflected in the blueprint and on the exam. Concepts and content are in paraphrased formats to allow broad coverage of the material and optimize study efforts.

The beginning sections of the workbook are devoted to enhancing knowledge and skills in the following areas:

- Exam process
- Study and testing techniques
- Calculator use

Content is designed to engage the analytical portions of the brain and help prepare you for the mathematical components of the exam.

From the introductory sections, the workbook progresses to individual areas on each of the seventeen CIH exam blueprint rubrics. These exam blueprint rubrics utilize the question and answer format designed to mimic the type of questions offered on the exam. The examination covers a tremendous amount of material; consideration has been given to the time commitment as explanations are offered to reduce additional research time.

The questions presented are representative of the questions found on the actual examination. For this reason, you must gain enough knowledge of areas to which the question is pertaining, which may require additional study. Repetition helps identify areas of strength and weakness, and closes knowledge gaps.

The assumption is that only fully qualified practitioners will attempt to sit for the CIH examination, which means everyone using this workbook has a fundamental knowledge in the Industrial Hygiene field. Given this assumption, no attempt has been made to provide a comprehensive text. The workbook is designed as a guide, and depending upon an individual's knowledge baseline, additional research may be required.

The challenge of achieving certification is a difficult task. Embrace the journey of professional development in preparation for the exam. The modern health and safety professional must be a dynamic, adaptive leader and lifelong learner.

This curriculum has been carefully checked for accuracy, but errors may exist. Should an error be discovered, contact the author via info@spansafetyworkshops.com

Overview of Certification Requirements:

Education, experience and examination are the foundations of ABIH-certification in industrial hygiene. The following information concerning the requirements for certification may have changed after publication. It is strongly suggested candidates contact the ABIH for current information.

Education qualification:
- A regionally accredited college or university, with a bachelor's degree in biology, chemistry, engineering, physics or an ABET accredited program in industrial hygiene or safety.
    - Other colleges and degrees will be considered by the Board.
    - The candidate must have academic or continuing education coursework specifically addressing ethics, industrial hygiene toxicology, fundamentals, measurements and controls.

Experience qualification:
- Best obtained through a relationship with a practicing Certified Industrial Hygienist (CIH).
- Therefore, several years of broad experience are necessary before a person may sit for the CIH examination.

Certification is a three-step process:
1. Eligibility
2. Preparation
3. Examination

Specifications for candidate eligibility can be found in the Candidate Handbook, which provides key information for education, experience, deadlines, Professional Reference Questionnaires (PRQ) and applications. Examinations are offered in spring and fall of each year at over 425 testing sites. Examinations are computer-based and scored as soon as the candidate has completed the examination.

IH Certification Process

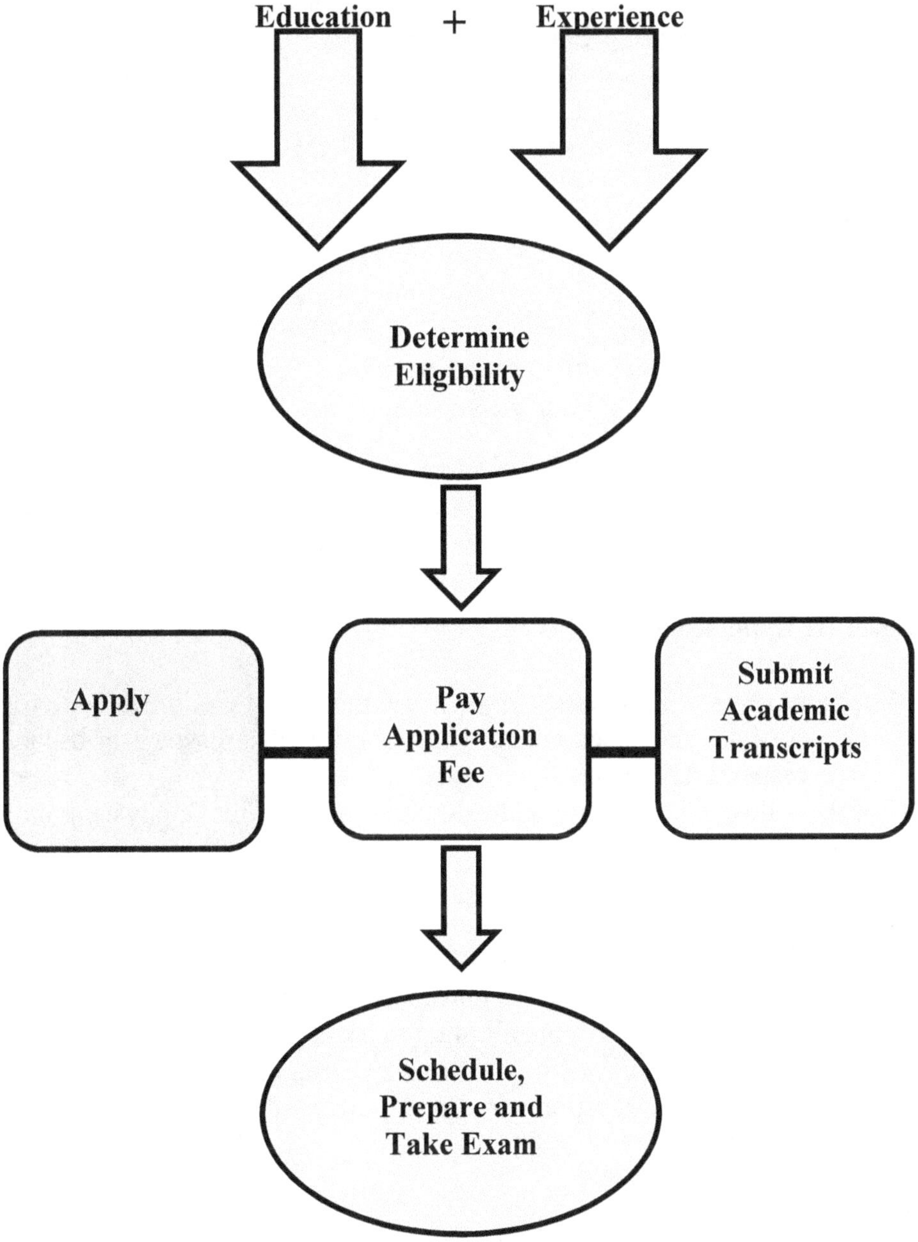

Eligibility

Possess at least a 4-year bachelor's degree from a regionally-accredited college or university:
- o Biology, Chemistry, Physics, or Engineering, or
- o IH or Safety from an ABET-accredited program,
- o With at least 60 semester hours of science, math, engineering, or science-based technology (15 hours at the junior, senior or graduate level).

Specific IH Course Work
- o Completed at least:
    - 180 academic contact hours* or 240 continuing education contact hours of IH coursework with at least half of those hours in the areas of Fundamentals of IH, Toxicology, Measurements and Controls
        - 1 semester credit hour = 15 academic hours; 1CEU = 10 continuing education hours
    - 2 hours of ethics training or coursework
- o The IH Coursework Document Form is accessible via ABIH.org, under the Document Library tab.

Professional Level IH Experience:
- o Completed at least:
    - 4 or more years of IH practice (1 year or 6 months of credit available for graduates of an ABET-accredited IH program, with a master's or bachelor's degree, respectively), and
    - 2 of the following occupational health stressors: chemical, physical, biological or ergonomics.

Professional References:
- o Provide at least 2 written confidential questionnaires from:
    - Current supervisor to verify your current level of IH work.
    - All other supervisors verifying all other work experience periods claimed.
    - One CIH who is familiar with your work experience.
- o The Professional Reference Questionnaire Form is accessible via ABIH.org, under the Document Library tab.

Application

Complete all of the following sections:
- o Application forms, fees, and deadlines.
- o College or university degree transcripts, including international degrees.
- o IH Related Courses Documentation Form.
- o Work experience documentation.
- o Professional References Questionnaires.
- o The Application Form is accessible via ABIH.org, under the Document Library tab.

Before taking the CIH Examination, an Application Form must be completed. There is a non-refundable **Application Fee** of $150 for the review. Mail the completed Application Form and Fee to the address provided on the form.

- o   Spring Exam (offered during April and May) due date: **February 1.**
- o   Fall Exam (offered during October and November) due date: **August 1.**

Official transcripts for your college or university degrees is required. They must show all degree courses and when they were completed. They must be sent directly to ABIH. If that's not possible, send official transcripts in a sealed envelope with the registrar's stamp across the seal. Document your IH-related courses by completing the IH Coursework Document Form. Documenting certificates for each course or stand-alone exam is required. Include all this information with your Application Form.

The applicant is required to provide work history for at least 4 years (48 months) at a professional IH level. One year or 6 months of credit is available for graduates of an ABET accredited IH program with a master's or bachelor's degree, respectively. Each reference must complete a Professional Reference Questionnaire and send it directly to ABIH. Two questionnaires are required; one from a current supervisor and one from a CIH who knows about your work.

Schedule and Take Exam

To obtain certification as a CIH, an examinee must:
- o   Submit a completed application and have it approved.
- o   Receive notice that he or she is approved to sit for the exam.
- o   Pay the examination fee of $350.
- o   Schedule the location and time of exam through the Prometric® website: www.prometric.com
- o   The Exam Scheduling Fact Sheet Form is accessible via ABIH.org, under the Document Library tab.
- o   Pass the exam.

The intended purpose of the exam is to ensure that professionals working in this field have the skills and knowledge identified as important in the practice of industrial hygiene.

Exams are offered electronically at Prometric® testing locations during two windows (April-May and October-November) each year. To locate a test center, log on to the Prometric® website and follow the instructions provided.

According to the American Board of Industrial Hygienist (ABIH), the table below states the percent of examinees who passed the exam from 2012 to 2017.

Exam Pass Rate 2012 – 2017

Year	Number of Examinees	Number of Participants Who Passed the Exam	Percent of Participants Who Passed the Exam
Spring 2017	286	139	48.6%
Fall 2016	270	117	43.3%
Spring 2016	252	124	49.2%
Fall 2015	269	132	49.1%
Spring 2015	251	136	54.2%
Fall 2014	285	108	37.9%
Spring 2014	257	108	42.0%
Fall 2013	279	106	38.0%
Spring 2013	253	126	49.8%
Fall 2012	269	128	47.6%
Spring 2012	257	93	36.2%

The Industrial Hygiene Professional

To perform professional functions, individuals practicing in the profession generally have education, training and experience from a common body of knowledge. They need to have a fundamental knowledge of physics; chemistry; biology; physiology; toxicology; statistics; mathematics; computer science; engineering mechanics; industrial processes; business; communication; and management. Many have backgrounds or advanced study in other disciplines, such as management and business administration, engineering, education, physical and social sciences. Others have advanced study in industrial hygiene, and this additional background extends their expertise beyond the basics of the profession.

Typical occupational settings are manufacturing; insurance; risk management; government; education; consulting; construction; healthcare; engineering and design; waste management; petroleum; facilities management; retail; transportation; and utilities. Within these contexts, professionals must adapt their functions to fit the mission, operations and climate of their employer. Not only must individuals in the profession acquire the knowledge and skills to perform these functions effectively in their employment context; they must also continue their education and training; stay current with new technologies, understand changes in laws and regulations, respond to changes in the workforce, workplace and world business, and remain current regarding political and social climates.

Professional Codes of Ethics and Standards of Conduct

Ethics is a rational reflection upon good and evil (without weighing in on the question of heaven or hell, angels and demons). The word *ethics* refers to our identification of the "good" in any given situation as well as the rationale for the identification.

Ethics engages each of us at the level of the reasoning process that goes into every decision we make, whether for our own happiness or that of another. Sound ethical judgment arises when proper habits of thought give way to confidence in the right conduct and in completing the appropriate action.

There are rigorous professional guidelines and regulations in place regarding ethics for an industrial hygiene professional. Below is a list of some of them:

- American Industrial Hygiene Association and American Conference of Governmental Industrial Hygienists Joint Ethical Principles
- American Board of Industrial Hygiene Code of Ethics
- Board of Certified Safety Professionals Code of Ethics and Professional Conduct
- American Society of Safety Engineers' Code of Professional Conduct
- International Code of Ethics for Occupational Health Professionals
- Federal Contractor Code of Business Ethics and Conduct (48 CFR 3.10)
- American Society of Civil Engineers Code of Ethics
- National Society of Professional Engineers Code of Ethics
- Institute of Hazardous Materials Management Code of Ethics

As a professional, you should be familiar with the codes of conduct pertinent to your work. However, in and of themselves, they are insufficient. You must also develop a robust code of personal ethics. The avoidance of wrong is not the same as doing right. Professionals must honor a high ethical standard that encompasses clients, colleagues and community. You must not only behave ethically; you must strive to encourage ethical behavior in others.

American Board of Industrial Hygiene Code of Ethics[1]

The American Board of Industrial Hygiene (ABIH) is a voluntary, non-profit, professional credentialing organization. ABIH certifies qualified industrial hygienists engaged in the practice of industrial hygiene who have met the professional knowledge standards established by the Board of Directors. Regardless of any other professional affiliation, the ABIH Code of Ethics (Code) applies to each individual certified by the ABIH as a Certified Industrial Hygienist (CIH) or a Certified Associate Industrial Hygienist (CAIH) (certificants), and each individual seeking ABIH certification (candidates). The Code serves as the *minimal* ethical standards for the professional behavior of ABIH certificants and candidates.

The Code is designed to provide appropriate ethical practice guidelines and enforceable standards of conduct for all certificants and candidates. The Code also serves as a professional resource for industrial hygienists and those served by ABIH certificants and candidates.

Preamble/General Guidelines

The ABIH is dedicated to the implementation of appropriate professional standards designed to serve the public, employees, employers, clients and the industrial hygiene profession. First and foremost, ABIH certificants and candidates give priority to health and safety interests related to the protection of people, and act in a manner that promotes integrity and reflects positively on the profession, and act in accordance with accepted moral, ethical and legal standards.

As professionals in the field of industrial hygiene, ABIH certificants and candidates have the obligation to maintain high standards of integrity and professional conduct; accept responsibility for their actions; continually seek to enhance their professional capabilities; practice with fairness and honesty; and encourage others to act in a professional manner consistent with the certification standards and responsibilities set forth below.

---

[1] Effective Date: May 25, 2007

I. Responsibilities to ABIH, the profession and the public.
A. Certificant and candidate compliance with all organizational rules, policies and legal requirements.

1. Comply with laws, regulations, policies and ethical standards governing professional practice of industrial hygiene and related activities.
2. Provide accurate and truthful representations concerning all certification and recertification information.
3. Maintain the security of ABIH examination information and materials, including the prevention of unauthorized disclosures of test information.
4. Cooperate with ABIH concerning ethics matters and the collection of information related to an ethics matter.
5. Report apparent violations of the ethics code by certificants and candidates upon a reasonable and clear factual basis.
6. Refrain from public behavior that is clearly in violation of professional, ethical or legal standards.

II. Responsibilities to clients, employers, employees and the public.
A. Education, experience, competency and performance of professional services.

1. Deliver competent services with objective and independent professional judgment in decision-making.

2. Recognize the limitations of one's professional ability and provide services only when qualified. The certificant/candidate is responsible for determining the limits of his/her own professional abilities based on education, knowledge, skills, practice experience and other relevant considerations.

3. Make a reasonable effort to provide appropriate professional referrals when unable to provide competent professional assistance.

4. Maintain and respect the confidentiality of sensitive information obtained in the course of professional activities unless the information is reasonably understood to pertain to unlawful activity; a court or governmental agency lawfully directs the release of the information; the client or the employer expressly authorizes the release of specific information; or the failure to release such information would likely result in death or serious physical harm to employees and/or the public.

5. Properly use professional credentials, and provide truthful and accurate representations concerning education, experience, competency and the performance of services.

6. Provide truthful and accurate representations to the public in advertising, public statements or representations, and in the preparation of estimates concerning costs, services and expected results.

7. Recognize and respect the intellectual property rights of others and act in an accurate, truthful and complete manner, including activities related to professional work and research.

8. Affix or authorize the use of one's ABIH seal, stamp or signature only when the document is prepared by the certificant/candidate or someone under his/her direction and control.

B. Conflict of interest and appearance of impropriety.

1. Disclose to clients' or employers' significant circumstances that could be construed as a conflict of interest or an appearance of impropriety.

2. Avoid conduct that could cause a conflict of interest with a client, employer, employee or the public.

3. Assure that a conflict of interest does not compromise legitimate interests of a client, employer, employee or the public and does not influence or interfere with professional judgments.

4. Refrain from offering or accepting significant payments, gifts or other forms of compensation or benefits in order to secure work or that are intended to influence professional judgment.

C. Public health and safety.

1. Follow appropriate health and safety procedures, in the course of performing professional duties, to protect clients, employers and employees.

Accredited Certification vs. Certificate Program

Accredited Certification	Certificate Program
Results from an assessment process	Results from an educational process
Typically requires some amount of professional experience	For novice and experienced professionals
Awarded by a third-party, standard-setting organization	Awarded by training and educational programs or institutions
Indicates master/competency as measured against a defensible set of standards, usually by application or exam	Indicates completion of a course or series of courses with a specific focus; is different than a degree granting program
Standards set through a defensible, industry-wide process (job analysis/role delineation) that results in an outline of required knowledge and skills	Course content set a variety of ways (faculty committee; dean; instructor; occasionally though defensible analysis of topic care)
Typically results in a designation to use after one's name; may result in a document to hang on the wall or keep in a wallet	Usually listed on a resume detailing education; may result in a document to hang on the wall
Has on-going requirements to maintain; individual must demonstrate knowledge of content; holder must demonstrate he/she continues to meet requirements	Is the end result; individual may or may not demonstrate knowledge of course content at the end of a set period in time

Benefits of Certification

The process of certification commands a considerable amount of effort. Many health & safety practitioners consider if the advantages of certification justify the effort. The primary advantage of certification is that it provides a credential. The CIH indicates that a health and safety professional has achieved a standard level of qualification as judged by their professional peers. This level of qualification is important in establishing credibility within the growing field of Environment, Safety and Health. As the health and safety community gains a greater understanding of the CIH certification, the employment opportunities will increase for personnel holding certification. Additionally, the demand for increased technicians for industrial hygiene monitoring and safety related duties has increased tremendously. This demand has made the CIH a unique "stand-alone" certification that provides increased status for health and safety practitioners. The CIH certification has maintained a high degree of credibility because of the affiliation with the ABIH.

The primary advantage of certification is that it provides a credential. The CIH indicates that a professional has achieved a standard level of qualification as judged by their professional peers. This level of qualification is important in establishing credibility within the growing field of Safety, Health and Environment (SH&E). Employment opportunities are much greater for personnel holding certification, and the courts recognize the certification as a step toward authentication as an expert witness. Certification is almost always required to practice consultant work in the field of occupational health and safety.

There are several reasons that should cause candidates to think about starting the process of obtaining certification *right now.*

- A growing trend by states to license safety professionals, much like physicians, engineers, architects and other professionals. Some states have that authority under their duty to "protect the health, safety and welfare of the public."
- Substantial support to modify existing safety and health laws to acknowledge certified "safety specialists and industrial hygienists". Some projects require a certified professional to be on staff.
- Certified professionals obtain employment earlier and receive greater compensation than non-certified employees.
- As the requirements increase, the examinations may become even more dynamic, complex, difficult to pass and expensive, both in time and financial investments.

These and other recent developments comprise a future environment where a certification is going to be the desired/required credential. Being a CIH will become much more important, more lucrative, and more difficult to obtain. Like the other professional certification/registration examinations, the CIH exams should be taken as early in one's career as possible.

Note: The following information concerning the requirements for certification may have changed after publication. We strongly suggest you contact the ABIH (www.abih.org) for current information.

The entire process of certification generally takes 3 to 6 months, thus allowing ample time to **PLAN** an individual study program. Costs associated with the certification process are as follows:

Table: CIH CRITERIA	
Minimum Education	A 4-year degree in Biology, Chemistry, Physics, OR Engineering, or IH or Safety from an ABET-accredited program, with at least 60 semester hours of science, math, engineering, or science-based technology (15 hours at the junior, senior or graduate level).
Training Prerequisite	N/A
Work Experience	4 years of professional practice
Application Fees	$150
Examination Fees	$350
Reapplication Fees	$75
Renewal Fees	$125
Recertification (5-year cycle)	40 points, with 10 IH and .33 ethics

The above information is accurate as of this printing. For more current information, candidates should contact the Board at www.abih.org.

Taking the Computer Based Exam

Testing on computer is done at Prometric® testing centers. Exams are offered electronically at Prometric® testing locations during two windows (April-May and October-November) each year. To locate a test center, log on to Prometric's website (Prometric.com) and follow the instructions provided. Schedule the location and time of the exam through the Prometric® website. An Exam Scheduling Fact Sheet Form is accessible via ABIH.org, found under the Document Library tab.

Prometric® is an Educational Testing Service (ETS) and a trusted provider of technology enabled testing and assessment solutions. It operates a secure network of 8,000 test centers in more than 160 countries, giving convenient access, as well as a wide selection of times and dates for testing, to test takers anywhere in the world. To contact Prometric®, visit their website and click on the Contact Us tab. Several options are listed on the page.

NO NOTES OR REFERENCE MATERIALS ARE ALLOWED
For worldwide locations, visit www.prometric.com.

About the Computer Exam

NOTE: The best and most current source of information on procedures and policies for the computer test is directly from ABIH at www.abih.org.

Question 1: *How do the questions appear on the computer screen? How do I make answer selections? Can I back up or mark questions so that I can come back to them?*
Answer: Examination questions appear one at a time and look very similar to the questions in the workbook. With a mouse or keys, the candidate selects the preferred answer and moves on to the next question. Since the computer test is user friendly, candidates do not have to be computer literate to take this exam.

Question 2: *Can I bring food or drinks into the exam room?*
Answer: No. All candidates are given a small locker for personal belongings, including snacks, purses, watches, etc. Access to this locker may or may not be allowed depending upon the testing center.

Question 3: *What can I take into the exam room?*
Answer: Only the approved calculators and ID cards are permitted. Everything else must go into personal lockers.

Question 4: *Are there any children in the exam room?*
Answer: No. The room is for adult testing only.

Question 5: *How many other people are in the room?*
Answer: There are multiple workstations in the exam room. The number of people varies with time and day. The proctor has a view of the entire room via glass window and corner mirrors on the ceiling. Testing is also taped by video and audio monitoring.

Question 6: *Can I take breaks?*
Answer: Yes, as many and as often as necessary. However, the clock keeps running and signing out is required each time, along with a finger print check. The examination is divided into two 90-minute sections, thus providing a convenient break opportunity.

Question 7: *Do I need IDs?*
Answer: One ID with photo and signature is mandatory. Photograph and a finger print are completed during sign-in.

Question 8: *Do I need to bring my authorization letter?*
Answer: This letter is usually not required, but it is advised to take it just in case.

Question 9: *Can I schedule the exam any time?*
Answer: No. Certain times are designated for professional exams. Book your testing slot several weeks in advance to secure the desired time and day.

Question 10: *Is there enough time to finish the exam?*
Answer: This is very subjective. Many candidates have found there was plenty of time to finish testing and have adequate review time, but other people did not finish in the allotted time.

Question 11: *Are there graphs to interpret? How clear are the graphics?*
Answer: Yes, there are a limited number of graphs to read. They are a slightly harder to read on the screen, but not significantly. Graphics are acceptable.

Question 12: *Are the math formulas provided?*
Answer: The formula sheet, ventilation plates and conversions are provided as a computer based reference at the examination.

Applied Study & Exam Techniques

The examination blueprint outlines how the items on an examination are distributed across domains and tasks/topics. Keys to success include the following:

1. Analyzing knowledge gaps and identify strengths and weaknesses
2. Designing a solid examination study plan
3. Developing test-taking strategies
4. Using the calculator properly

Converting your subject strengths and weaknesses into a study plan is likely to increase your overall examination score. Scoring well in one subject area can compensate for a weaker score in another subject area. However, there may not be enough items in your strong areas to achieve a passing score.

Note that knowledge and understanding are essential in passing the examination. Relying only on simulated examination items is not the best way to increase knowledge and understanding. Use simulated items to provide insight into the areas in which you should engage in additional study.

How to take the test

Knowing *how* to take the examination will help improve your score. The examination uses multiple-choice items with only one correct answer and three incorrect answers. The goal is to get as many items correct as possible; there is no penalty for selecting an incorrect answer. However, only correct answers count toward reaching the passing score. Below are strategies for test-taking.

- **Read the items carefully.**
  - o Psychometricians design multiple choice questions so that all the possible answer choices are plausible. Use deductive and inductive reasoning to eliminate detractor answer choices.
- **Understand the problem.**
  - o Consider the context
  - o What is given? What is wanted?
- **Use examination time wisely.**
  - o Conduct multiple passes solving the "easy" problems first and saving the challenging problems for the end.
- **Complete all items.**
  - o Blank answers are scored as wrong answers.

Preparing for the test

While studying resources, identify main thoughts or themes in the literature review. Draw on your experience and on professional and study references, and rewrite important ideas in your own words to help you remember the concepts in context. Additional references are listed later in the workbook.

In establishing a good study regiment, it is important to find a place conducive to studying. A good study area should meet the following criteria:

- The study place should be chosen exclusively for the purpose of studying. Avoid using a garage, workshop, family room or other area that represents recreation or other distractions. Find a location that represents a study island, where study is the **only** activity.
- Selected study area should have good lighting, ventilation, be temperature controlled, comfortable and quiet.
- A large table or desk to spread necessary readily available study and reference materials is a must. The purpose is to dedicate a comfortable, personal space with minimal interruptions.

Minimizing distractions

Securing a good place to study should eliminate as many external distractions as possible. Also, candidates should consider how to minimize internal distractions. Total elimination of external distractions is often possible; however, total elimination of internal distractions is nearly impossible and can only be minimized through focused thought.

Helpful hints for focusing the mind for studying include the following:

1. **Set realistic time limits, determining what to study and keeping with a schedule.** Studying a subject too long at one time can lead to daydreaming which reduces study effectiveness.
2. **Personal factors can be distracters and result in additional frustration.** All efforts should be attempted in avoiding personal issues. Rescheduling the CIH test date may be a consideration if serious personal problems exist.
3. **Minimize dealing with outside details**. Having too many obligations and/or responsibilities enables "brain creep". Consider keeping a notebook in the study area and jotting down appointments and details of projects as these brainstorms appear. It's impossible to totally prevent these details from surfacing, but by documenting them, it may free the mind to resume studies.

4. Be physically and mentally prepared to study.

- *Eat a well-balanced diet.* Increase protein intake; a proper level of blood sugar enhances studying effectiveness.
- *Get plenty of sleep.* Establish and maintain a regular work/rest cycle.
- *Exercise is beneficial for more than just an exam preparation.* Consider choosing a form of exercise that provides enjoyment and relaxation.
- *Avoid mental fatigue.* Allocate down time for breaks. The average supervisor should study for the CIH exam for two to four weeks. DO NOT attempt to cram overnight.

This section is designed to assist with mastering a learning methodology. This workbook uses a **Question & Answer** format to allow candidates to concentrate on areas that are unfamiliar and avoid over studying material in areas where the candidate already possesses enough knowledge to pass the exam.

The research has been completed by the authors, who have actually taken the exam, and researched the blueprint areas of interest to develop targeted learning outcomes. This allows candidates to determine if their current level knowledge is adequate, or if a more in-depth understanding is required.

Fundamental to this technique is a good core of questions. The technique is intended to be useful to practitioners who have mastered the skills and tasks necessary to perform in the safety and health arena.

How to use this workbook

When utilizing this workbook properly, the authors believe candidates can master areas necessary to achieve the goal of passing the CIH examination with minimum effort on research and actual study. The technique also has some very beneficial side effects. Candidates will find that the learning process enhances skill sets in becoming an improved and more proficient safety and health practitioner.

The process assumes candidates have the discipline to do the research and study the material where deficiencies may exist. Attempting to study using only the material presented in this workbook becomes a risk for not being adequately prepared for the examination.

Steps to using the **Question and Answer** (Q&A) method:

1. **Dead reckoning:** Use existing knowledge, experience, and test taking strategies; attempt to answer the question.

2. **Process check:** Review the results of each practice session and then study the explanation.

3. **Validate knowledge:** Was this a known or an unknown concept? Is the answer achieved with current knowledge base or the correct answer achieved by an educated guess or dumb luck? Note: This is a critical step in the Q&A learning process and determines if one can proceed or needs to gain more knowledge on the subject.

4. **Filter:** Move on or take notes. When comfortable with knowledge on the subject, move on to the next question. However, if the current level of knowledge on the subject or other aspects of the subject feels inadequate, then take additional notes about the information that is needed. The authors recommend candidates write in the workbook margins right next to the question.

5. **Enhance deficiencies:** Research and study deficient knowledge areas. After completing a set of questions and writing notes on information to study, a knowledge deficiency study plan can be developed. Research and study the material necessary to enhance the required knowledge. The authors advise focusing on notes in the workbook and staying on subject. It is very easy to wander into some other interesting subject and lose sight of the desired learning outcome. Keep the goal in mind to pass the test the first time.

How far into the topic does a student need to explore? The level of detail in the example question may serve as a representative indicator. Beyond the basics, another key indicator is the repetition of the workbook question. Content frequently appearing with only minor changes in question format indicates that the subject matter is important, and the authors anticipate the actual exam will have several questions dealing with that subject.

The Q&A method of studying is a proven method. The basic outline is delivered with questions, and students can then determine individual levels of subject knowledge. When additional knowledge is required, they can conduct more research and study to develop the required knowledge or skill. This learning technique has proven to be successful for many different levels of adult learners because **the individual** determines what material to study.

Please contact the authors at info@spansafetyworkshops.com with any questions or feedback on these study materials.

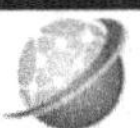
<h1>CIH Exam Study Workbook Volume I</h1>

Select Study References for the CIH Exam

<u>AIHA and ACGIH maintain lists of examination references for certification. Examination items are not necessarily taken directly from these sources. However, the information is relevant to the examination process.</u>

Anna, Daniel H. The Occupational Environment: Its Evaluation, Control and Management. Fairfax, VA: American Industrial Hygiene Association, 2011. Print.

ANSI/ASSE Z10 (2012). American National Standard for Occupational Health & Safety Management Systems. Des Plaines, Illinois: American Society of Safety Engineers. Print.

Bingham, Eula, Barbara Cohrssen, and F. A. Patty. Patty's Toxicology. Hoboken, NJ: Wiley, A John Wiley & Sons, 2012. Print.

Brown, Theodore L., Bruce Edward. Bursten, and LeMay, Harold. Chemistry: The Central Science. Upper Saddle River: Prentice-Hall International, 2000. Print.

Burton, D. J. Industrial Hygiene Workbook: The Occupational Health Sciences. Bountiful, UT: Carr Printing, 2003. Print.

ABIH. American Board of Industrial Hygiene. Web.

ACGIH Industrial Ventilation Handbook, Manual of Recommended Practices, American Conference of Governmental Industrial Hygienists.

ACGIH, Threshold Limit Values and Biological Exposure Indices.

Engelhardt, Susan J., Judith M. Grunewald, Ralph Grunewald, Dee A. Kaiser, and Joshua P. Walkowicz. Radiation Protection: A Practical Guide. Print.

EPA. United States Environmental Protection Agency. Web.

Fleeger, Allan K., and Dean R. Lillquist. Industrial Hygiene Reference & Study Guide. Fairfax, VA: American Industrial Hygiene Association, 2011. Print.

Hathaway, Gloria J., Nick H. Proctor, James P. Hughes, and Michael L. Fischman. Proctor and Hughes' Chemical Hazards of the Workplace. 3rd ed. Print.

Jahn, Steven D., William H. Bullock, and Joselito S. Ignacio. A Strategy for Assessing and Managing Occupational Exposures. Fairfax, VA: AIHA, 2015. Print.

Klaassen, Curtis D., Toxicology, The Basic Science of Poisons, Casarett and Doull's, 7th ed. Print.

NIOSH. The National Institute for Occupational Safety and Health. Centers for Disease Control and Prevention. Web.

OSHA. Occupational Safety and Health Administration. United States Department of Labor. Web.

Pagano, Marcello. Principles of Biostatistics. 2nd ed. Pacific Grove: Brooks/Cole, 2012. Print.

Plog, Barbara A., and Patricia Quinlan. Fundamentals of Industrial Hygiene. Itasca: National Safety Council, 2012. Print.

Stern, M.B, and S.Z Mansdorf. Applications and Computational Elements of Industrial Hygiene. Boca Raton,FL: Lewis, 1999. Print.

Stewart, James et al, Industrial Hygiene Calculations: A Professional Reference. Millennium Publishing. Print.

*The purpose of our exam study workbook is to guide your study effort in a focused direction by effectively streamlining the enormous amount of test material that could be presented. The best approach is to study the **right** material; specifically, the right reference material. Finding the right books from which to study is probably the most important single element in developing a personal study plan. SPAN is the curator of an impressive reference library from which the curriculum is developed. A more extensive list of references is located at the back of the workbook.*

The CIH Exam Blueprint

The examination blueprint is based on surveys of what professionals do in practice. The CIH examination is required for candidates to demonstrate knowledge of professional practice at the CIH level. The top levels, called rubrics, represent the major functions performed by professionals at the CIH level. Each rubric contains several topics of knowledge and skills.

CIH Blueprint

Rubric 1:	Air Sampling and Instrumentation
Rubric 2:	Analytical Chemistry
Rubric 3:	Basic Science
Rubric 4:	Biohazards
Rubric 5:	Biostatistics and Epidemiology
Rubric 6:	Community Exposure
Rubric 7:	Engineering Controls – Ventilation, Radiation, Noise, Heat
Rubric 8:	Ergonomics
Rubric 9:	Health Risk Analysis and Hazard Communication
Rubric 10:	Industrial Hygiene Program Management
Rubric 11:	Noise
Rubric 12:	Non-Engineering Control
Rubric 13:	Radiation – Ionizing
Rubric 14:	Radiation – Non-Ionizing
Rubric 15:	Thermal Stressors
Rubric 16:	Toxicology
Rubric 17:	Work Environment and Industrial Processes

The CIH certification exam is designed to measure the broad spectrum of knowledge required in professional practice. Accordingly, many questions on the application of science, engineering and professional practice will be encountered.

Questions about the pass rate, passing score, standard deviation, etc., should be addressed to the American Board of Industrial Hygiene. www.abih.org

Rubric 1: Air Sampling and Instrumentation

Selection, use and limitations of:
- Field air-sampling instruments
- Full-shift and grab samples, including direct reading instruments

Set-up, calibration and use of:
- Air-sampling apparatus
- Direct-reading instruments

Sampling strategy considerations
Calculations related to sampling and calibration

Rubric 2: Analytical Chemistry

Laboratory analytical procedures and calculations for work place environmental samples:
- Gas chromatography
- Infrared, visible and ultraviolet spectrophotometry
- High performance liquid chromatography
- Mass spectroscopy
- Atomic absorption spectrophotometry
- Wet-chemical methods
- Microscopy and laboratory quality assurance
- Chain of custody

Rubric 3: Basic Science

General scientific concepts:
- Chemistry
- Biochemistry
- Biology
- Anatomy
- Physiology
- General physics
- Mathematics

Properties of:
- Flammable materials
- Combustible materials
- Reactive materials

Calculations relative to:
- Gas laws
- Airborne concentrations
- Unit of measure conversions
- Conditions of non-standard pressure

Rubric 4: Biohazards

Principles of:
- Sanitation
- Personal Hygiene

Set-up. calibration and use of:
- Air-sampling apparatus
- Direct-reading instruments

The recognition, evaluation and control of biohazards, including:
- Viruses
- Bacteria
- Molds
- Allergens
- Toxins
- Recombinant products
- Bloodborne pathogens

Infectious diseases that appear in workplaces, including:
- Industry
- Agriculture
- Homes
- Offices
- Health care facilities

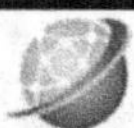

Rubric 5: Biostatistics and Epidemiology

Principles of epidemiology
- Techniques to study the distribution of occupationally induced diseases and physiological conditions in workplaces, and the factors that influence their frequency
- Concepts of prospective and retrospective studies
- Morbidity and mortality
- Animal experimentation studies
- Data and distribution of data
- Basic biostatistics
- Statistical and non-statistical interpretation of data in the evaluation of hazards

Rubric 6: Community Exposure

Areas of study include:
- Air pollution and air cleaning technology
- Ambient air-quality considerations
- Emission source sampling
- Atmospheric dispersion of pollutants
- Ambient air monitoring

Health and environmental effect of air pollutants and related calculations, including:
- Emergency response and planning
- Water pollution
- Hazardous waste
- Environmental fate and transport

Rubric 7: Engineering Controls-Ventilation

Controls of chemical and physical exposures through engineering measures, such as local exhaust ventilation, dilution ventilation, isolation, containment and process change.
Mechanics and related calculations of:
- Airflow
- Ventilation measurements
- Design principles
- In-plant recirculation air-cleaning technology

Engineering control of:
- Noise sources
- Ionizing and non-ionizing radiation
- Thermal stressors
- Vibration sources

Rubric 8: Ergonomics

Application of principles from:
- Anthropometry
- Human factors engineering
- Biomechanics
- Work physiology
- Human anatomy
- Occupation medicine and facilities engineering to design and organize the workplace in order to prevent injuries and illnesses.

Rubric 9: Health Risk Analysis and Hazard Communication

Understanding principles and requirements for the interpretation and use of guidelines for the assessment of health hazards, including:
- American Conference of Governmental Industrial Hygienists (ACGIH)
  - Threshold Limit Values (TLVs)
  - Biological Exposure Indices (BEIs)
  - Industrial Ventilation Guidelines
- American National Standards Institute (ANSI) standards
- American Society for Heating, Refrigeration, and Air Conditioning Engineers (ASHRAE) guidelines
- American Society for Testing and Materials (ASTM) standards

Understanding the risk reduction process, including:
- The hierarchy of controls
- Control banding
- Hazard communication
- Training of employees
- Communication of recommendations by appropriate techniques to implement control actions

---

Rubric 10: Industrial Hygiene Program Management

Acquisition, allocation and control of resources to accomplish industrial hygiene objectives of anticipation, recognition, evaluation and control in a timely and effective manner.
Topics include:
- Auditing
- Investigation methods
- Data management and integration
- Establishment of policy
- Planning
- Delegation of authority
- Accountability
- Risk communication
- Organizational structure
- Decision making
- ABIH Code of Ethics

Rubric 11: Noise

- The health effects resulting from exposure to noise and vibration
- Calculations related to combining noise sources and octave band measurements
- Audiometric testing programs
- Exposure measurement, evaluation and control

Rubric 12: Non-Engineering Controls

Personal protective equipment:
- Principles governing selection
- Use and limitations of respirators and protective clothing
- Respirator fit-testing
- Breathing air specifications
- Glove permeability
- Eye protection
- Use of administrative controls

Rubric 13: Radiation - Ionizing

The physical/source characteristics. Health and biological effects associated with:
- Alpha
- Beta
- Gamma
- Neutron
- X-radiation
- Exposure measurement, evaluation and control

Rubric 14: Radiation – Non-Ionizing

The physical characteristics and health effects associated with:
- Electromagnetic fields
- Static, electric and magnetic fields
- Lasers
- Radiofrequency
- Microwaves
- Ultraviolet
- Visible
- Infrared and illumination
- Exposure measurement, evaluation and control

Rubric 15: Thermal Stressors

Adverse health effects associated with:
- Heat and cold
- Symptoms of temperature related health effects
- Exposure control techniques
- First aid/medical response

Rubric 16: Toxicology

The health effects resulting from exposure to chemical substances, including:
- Single agents
- Mixtures
- Natural and synthetic agents

Other study areas include:
- Symptomatology
- Pharmacokinetics
- Mode of action
- Additive, synergistic and antagonistic effects
- Routes of entry
- Absorption, metabolism and excretion
- Target organs
- Toxicity testing protocols
- Aerosol deposition
- Respiratory tract clearance
- Carcinogenic, mutagenic, teratogenic and reproductive hazards

Rubric 17: Work Environments and Industrial Processes

The hazards associated with specific industrial or manufacturing processes.
Topics include:
- Confined space entry
- Spray-painting
- Welding
- Abrasive-blasting
- Vapor-degreasing
- Foundry operations
- Hazardous waste site remediation
- General indoor environmental issues

CIH Calculator Math Review

To successfully complete the exam, the certificant must master the basic functions of a scientific calculator.

Conversions and Formula Transpositions are an important part of the process used in solving many of the problems encountered on the exam; several pages are devoted to this process.

Calculations provide examples of the complexity historically encountered in the CIH examinations. You will find solutions to all problems immediately following each section.

Select an Approved Calculator

The CIH exams require the use of a good scientific calculator. Those taking the CIH examination will be allowed to bring one or two calculators into the secure examination facility; any calculator brought into the examination must be on the approved list on the Board for Global EHS Credentialing web page.

Make sure you know how to use your calculator(s) so you don't waste valuable time trying to understand how to use it once the examination clock starts. It is a good idea to practice working solutions and to be able to recall the correct calculator procedures.

Calculator Practice Questions

Solve the following using an ABIH approved calculator.
Note: Rounding of numbers for the examination is not a problem. Due to the differences in calculator accuracy, the test will use approximate answers that will not be affected by reasonable rounding errors

1)   Calculate $69.95 - 10\%$ discount =...________

2)   Calculate 14×356...________

3)   Calculate $\pi \times 3.6^2$ ....________

4)   Calculate $\dfrac{\left(\frac{1}{2} \times 6^2\right)}{\sqrt{9}}$ ....________

5)   Calculate $5^{4.87}$ ....________

6)   Calculate $\sqrt[4.87]{2535}$ ....________

7)   Calculate $\log 15.32$...________

8)   Calculate $90 + 16.61 \times \log_{10} 2$ ....________

9)   Calculate $1 - e^{-2.5}$..________

10)   Calculate 45^{-1} ....________

11) Calculate $\dfrac{1}{45}$ ....________

12) Calculate $(64)^{1/2}$ ....________

13) Calculate sine 30 ....________

14) Calculate arcsine of 0.5 ....________

15) Calculate $\dfrac{(4\times5)}{(5\times4)}$ ....________

16) Calculate $\dfrac{\frac{70+50}{12}}{5\times5}$ ....________

17) Calculate $\sqrt{4.5\times2}$ ....________

Calculator Solutions

1.   Calculate $69.95 - 10% discount = ...$62.96

2.   Calculate 14×356 4984

3.   Calculate $\pi \times 3.6^2$ 40.72

4.   Calculate $\dfrac{\left(\frac{1}{2} \times 6^2\right)}{\sqrt{9}}$ 6

5.   Calculate $5^{4.87}$ 2535

6.   Calculate $\sqrt[4.87]{2535}$ 5

7.   Calculate $\log 15.32$ 1.19

8.   Calculate $90 + 16.61 \times \log_{10} 2$ 95

9.   Calculate $1 - e^{-2.5}$ 0.92

10.   Calculate 45^{-1} 0.022

11.   Calculate $\dfrac{1}{45}$ 0.022

12.   Calculate $(64)^{1/2}$ 8

13.   Calculate $\text{sine } 30$ 0.5

14.   Calculate arcsine of 0.5 30

15.   Calculate $\dfrac{(4 \times 5)}{(5 \times 4)}$ 1

16.   Calculate $\dfrac{\frac{70 + 50}{12}}{5 \times 5}$ 0.4

17.   Calculate $\sqrt{4.5 \times 2}$ 3

Rubric 1: Air Sampling and Instrumentation

Air sampling is used to evaluate employee exposure, assist in the design or evaluation of control measures, and document compliance with government regulations. Inhalation hazards shall be evaluated and controlled by comparing the measured concentration of an airborne chemical to a recognized exposure limit. Methods for air sample collection have been developed to ensure that accurate and meaningful information is collected.

Two approaches are generally practiced when selecting a population or group to conduct air sampling. The first approach focuses on a population that performs routine, daily tasks. The second approach focuses on a population that has the highest potential for exposure during a work process. Once the air sampling population is defined, the air sampling methodology has to be determined. Two options are practical for determining the air sampling methodology. The first option is conducting air sampling for a homogeneous exposure group (HEG). HEG is defined as workers doing a specific job with a similar task, and the overall exposure profile is similar. The second option is conducting air sampling on employees who are randomly selected from all the workers in the group. The random approach provides a statistically relevant result.

Before the air sampling process begins, the instrument(s) must first be calibrated. The calibration process is a comparison between one instrument's response and a reference instrument of known response and known accuracy. The quality of the calibrator used or referenced is essential to determine the overall quality of the calibration process.

There are two general categories for air sampling instrumentation:
- **Direct reading instruments**
  - Direct reading instruments provide an instantaneous measurement of concentration and can also be used to display the variation in concentration throughout the duration of the sampling period.
- **Sample collection devices**
  - Sampling collection devices pull air through media at a known flow rate for the duration of the sampling period. After the sampling period is complete, the media is sent to an accredited laboratory for appropriate analysis.

Topics covered include information about sample strategies, selection, calibration, use and limitations of air sampling equipment. In addition, calculations related to sampling and calibration are addressed.

Important Terms and Concepts

Absorption- Gas or vapor passes through liquid collection media. Gas is absorbed in the liquid and then analyzed by wet chemistry or automated method.

Adsorption- A surface collection mechanism. Gas or vapor adheres (absorbs) to the surface of the collection media.

Calibration- The process of comparing one instriment's response to that of a reference instrument of known response and known accuracy.

Dusts- Dry particle aerosols produced by mechanical processes, such as breaking, grinding and pulverizing.

Fibers- Elongated particles having an aspect ratio (length/width) of greater than 3:1.

Fogs- Droplet aerosols produced by condensation.

Fumes- Very fine solid aerosol particles produced from vaporized solids.

Gas- Formless fluid that expands to occupy the entire space in which it is confined. Material is normally a gas at standard temperature and pressure (STP). Requires increased pressure and decreased temperature to convert it to a liquid or solid.

Homogeneous Exposure Group- A group of employees who experience agent exposures similar enough that monitoring the agent exposures of any worker in the group provides data useful for predicting exposures to the remaining workers. The categorization of workers into these groups often involves categorization by process, job description and agents, although finer separation can be attained by further dividing on the basis of task analysis. Abbreviated HEG. Modern literature uses the term similar exposure group (SEG).

Isokinetic Sampling- A representative sample independent of particulate size. Used for dust and particle measurements in power plants, furnaces, kilns, scrubbers, and in ambient air pollution measurements.

Mists- Spherical droplet aerosols produced by mechanical processes, such as spraying, splashing or bubbling.

Monodisperse- Composed of airborne particulates with a single size or a small range of sizes.

Particulate Matter- Fine or solid liquid particles, such as dust, fog, mist, smoke or sprays.

Micrometer- one micrometer (μm) is 1/1,000 millimeter. This is the common unit of measure for particulate matter.

Passive Monitor- Device that collects airborne gases and vapors at a rate controlled by a physical process, such as diffusion through a static air layer, or permeation through a membrane without the active movement of air through an air sampler.

Polydisperse- Composed of airborne particulates of many different sizes.

Smokes- A mixture of solid and liquid aerosol particle gasses and vapors resulting from incomplete combustion.

Vapor- A gaseous form of a material that is normally a liquid (or a solid) at standard temperature and pressure (STP). Becomes airborne (gaseous) through evaporation or sublimation. Can be converted to a liquid or solid through increased pressure or decreased temperature.

Particle Sampling and Deposition in the Lung

- **Inhalable Fraction-** Larger particles (50% cut-point at 100 µm) deposited in the nasopharyngeal region.
- **Thoracic Fraction-** Smaller particles (50% cut point at 10µm) deposited in the tracheobronchial region.
- **Respirable Fraction-** Smallest particles (50% cut point at 4µm) deposited in the pulmonary/alveolar region.

Particle size sampling is based on sedimentation techniques or impaction techniques. Sedimentation utilizes a cyclone that has a set cut-point based on a specified flow rate. Impaction methods include single stage and cascade impactors.

There are also direct reading particle measuring devices that provide real time particle concentration readings.

Table 1.1 PARTICULATE SUMMARY	
Dust	Dry particle aerosols produced by mechanical processes, such as breaking, grinding and pulverizing.
Fumes	Very fine solid aerosol particles produced from vaporized solids.
Mists	Spherical droplet aerosols produced by mechanical processes, such as spraying, splashing or bubbling.
Fogs	Droplet aerosols produced by condensation.
Smokes	A mixture of solid and liquid aerosol particle gasses and vapors resulting from incomplete combustion.
Fibers	Elongated particles having an aspect ratio (length/width) of greater than 3:1.

Gas and Vapor Sampling

Gas and vapor sampling can be performed with adsorbing media, absorbing media, evacuated cylinders, gas bags and direct reading instrumentation.

Absorption methods include the fritted bubbler and midget impinger. The vapor or gas is absorbed into the collection media (liquid) and then analyzed with wet chemistry techniques. These methods are subject to collection liquid spillage and device breakage.

Adsorption methods include charcoal tubes for non-polar organics, silica gel tubes for polar organics, and specialty tubes (Tenax, Cromsorb, etc.) for other compounds.

Evacuated cylinders (Summa cans) are rigid containers with a negative internal pressure and a flow regulating valve. The cylinder collects every vapor or gas in the air over a designated period of time (grab or full shift). The sample can then be analyzed for numerous contaminants that may have different laboratory analysis methods.

Bag sampling uses a pump to fill a mylar, tedlar or other chemically resistant bag. The period can be short (grab) or full shift. A limitation of this method is potential permeability of the bag.

Direct reading devices include colorimetric tubes, broad spectrum analyzers and specific gas monitors.

Colorimetric tubes are used for screening or grab sampling. The results are provided in real time. The chemical contaminant reacts with the sample media and produces a color change that is proportional to the concentration of the airborne contaminant. The tubes are simple, low cost and intrinsically safe. Their limitations include accuracy of reading by user and interferences from other chemicals.

Photoionization Detectors (PID) draw air into the device and expose the air to UV light. If the chemical has an ionization potential below the energy of the light, then it will be ionized and generate an electronic signal proportional to the chemical concentration. The signal is not specific to one chemical, but to all chemicals in the sample with ionization potential less than the light energy.

Gas detectors that utilize electrolytic cells or sensors are considered specific gas monitors. The sensors are electrochemical polarographic cells with a thin film on front. The detectors collect contaminants by either pumping or diffusion. When the specified chemical is detected, an electronic signal is generated.

Infrared monitors such as Miran use the absorption of infrared energy in specific energy bands that are unique to a specific chemical. The infrared detectors are subject to interference from other chemicals.

Approaches to Sampling

Integrated Sampling- Collecting samples continuously over the time period of the expected exposure.

Active Sampling- Using a sample pump to draw air through the collection media at a known flow rate. Usually performed according to NIOSH or OSHA methods that prescribe flow rates, volumes, media, shipping and handling techniques.

Passive Sampling- Allowing the gas or vapor to naturally diffuse into the collection media.

Passive Monitors - Collect chemical contaminants at a rate controlled by diffusion through a static layer of air or permeation through a membrane.

Passive monitor operation is based on the Diffusion Theory, which states the molecules will move along a concentration gradient from higher to lower. The underlying force of the movement is Brownian motion. Brownian motion is the random motion of particles suspended in a fluid (a liquid or a gas) resulting from their collision with the quick atoms or molecules in the gas or liquid. Fick's First Law of Diffusion defines the parameters of passive collection devices.

Fick's First Law of Diffusion

$$W = D\,(A/L)(C_1 - C_0)$$

Where:
W is the mass transfer rate (ng/sec).
D is the diffusion coefficient (cm^2/sec).
A is the cross-sectional area of the diffusion path (cm^2).
L is the length of the diffusion path (cm).
C_1 is the ambient concentration of the contaminant (ng/cm^3).
C_0 is the concentration of the contaminant at the collection surface (ng/m^3).

Air Sampling and Calibration

Air flow calibration will use primary or secondary calibration devices.

Primary devices use the internal volume of the device to measure air flow. They are accurate to $\pm$ 1% and are not effected by temperature or pressure changes. Primary flow rate meters include frictionless piston meters such as bubble meters or graphite pistons, spirometers and Marriotti Bottles. Spirometers measure displaced air over a given volumetric dimension, and Marriotti Bottles measure displaced water over a give volumetric dimension.

Secondary devices use something other than the internal volume of the device to measure air flow. They are accurate to $\pm$ 5%. An example of a secondary device is the rotameter, which is a variable air meter.

Accurate air sample volumes are necessary to obtain accurate indications of exposure concentrations. If the air flow is accurate, then the calculated volumes are correct.

Sample pumps must be calibrated prior to and after the sample. The pre-sample calibration and post-sample calibration can be used to determine the % error and then decide how to use the information based on recommended guidelines.

　

Rotameter Correction

$$Q_{actual}=Q_{indicated}\left(\frac{T_{act}}{T_{cal}} \; x \; \frac{P_{cal}}{P_{act}}\right)^{1/2}$$

Where:

Q_{actual} is the flow rate determined by field pressure and temperature corrections to the indicated flow rate.

$Q_{indicated}$ is the flow rate measured under field conditions.

T_{act} is the absolute temperature for field conditions.

T_{cal} is the absolute temperature for calibration conditions.

P_{act} is the absolute pressure for field conditions.

P_{cal} is the absolute pressure for calibrations conditions.

Use:

To correct flow rate for rotameter readings at T and P readings that are different from the calibration readings.

Example:

A rotameter is calibrated in Denver (P = 640 mm HG and T = 21 C) and is used in New Orleans (T = 18 C). The indicated flow rate was 2 L/m. What was sample volume collected over a 7 hour and 35-minute period?

$$\text{Equation 1.3} \quad Q_{actual}=Q_{indicated}\left(\frac{T_{act}}{T_{cal}} \; x \; \frac{P_{cal}}{P_{act}}\right)^{1/2}$$

$$Q_{actual}=2\left(\frac{18+273}{21+273} \; x \; \frac{640}{760}\right)^{1/2}$$

Note: The 760 is pressure at sea level

$$Q = 1.83 \text{ L/m}$$

$$FR \; x \; T = V$$
$$1.83 \text{ L/m x } 455 \text{ min} = 831 \text{ L}$$

Sampling Strategies

The first question to answer is "Why perform exposure monitoring?".
- Estimate worker exposure
- Determine compliance with standards or guidelines
- Determine effectiveness of controls
- Characterize emissions for establishing regulated areas or other reasons

Other questions to answer include the following:
- Is there a method?
- Who to sample?
- When to sample?
- How often to sample?
- What will be done with the information gained from the samples?

The following information is a general overview of the exposure assessment strategy process.
- **Develop a strategy**: Describe the approach and define what is an acceptable exposure.
- **Basic characterization**: Assemble information of processes, potential exposures and the work force.
- **Exposure assessment**: Assess exposures. Outcomes include 1) Grouping workers based on exposure profiles (SEGs); 2) Defining the exposure profile for each SEG relative to the exposure limit; 3) Using professional judgement about the acceptability of exposure for each profile.
- **Additional information gathering**: Prioritize additional monitoring or information gathering to aid in resolving uncertain exposure judgements.
- **Health hazard control:** Prioritize and utilize control strategies for unacceptable exposures.
- **Reassessment:** Re-evaluate exposures periodically. The frequency of reassessment should be defined based on the initial assessment results and/or changes in the process.
- **Communicate and document**: The results of the exposure assessment must be communicated. The results must be retained for compliance and program management purposes.

Rubric 1: Air Sampling and Instrumentation Questions

1. The gas or vapor passes through a liquid and is captured. The gas or vapor can be soluble and non-reactive with the liquid, or the liquid can contain a reactive reagent. This best describes what extraction technique?

   A) Adsorption.
   B) Desorption.
   C) Absorption.
   D) Degradation.

2. The laboratory chemist informs you that the limit of detection for acetic acid is 0.01 mg. You anticipate the concentration is $1/10^{th}$ of the exposure limit based on historical grab sample results. The exposure limit for acetic acid is 25 mg/m^3. What is the minimum sample volume required and the sample duration necessary to collect this volume if the pump is calibrated at 0.1 L/m.?

   A) 4 liters, 40 minutes.
   B) 0.4 liters, 4 minutes.
   C) 400 liters, 4000 minutes.
   D) 40 liters, 400 minutes.

3. All of the following are acceptable uses of area sampling except:

   A) Evaluate background concentrations.
   B) For compliance with a PEL or TLV.
   C) Locate sources of exposure.
   D) Evaluate the effectiveness of controls.

4. An IH trained in phase contrast microscopy is analyzing a filter for asbestos fiber density on the filter. Calculating the fiber density is the first of a two-step method for determining the airborne fiber concentration. If the fiber density is greater than 1300 f/mm^2, the results are reported as uncountable or probably biased. The sample for asbestos was collected over 450 minutes of an 8-hour shift at 2 L/m. After counting 100 fields, the average fiber count is 3 fibers per field. The field blank contains 0.01 fibers per field. It is known that the area of a 25 mm filter is 385 mm^2 and that the area of a graticule field is approximately 0.00785 mm^2. What is the fiber density, and is the sample acceptable?

   A) 1400 f/mm^2 and not acceptable.
   B) 381 f/mm^2 and acceptable.
   C) 3 f/mm^2 and not acceptable.
   D) 242 f/mm^2 and acceptable.

5. Another name for passive sampler is:

    A) Elutriator.
    B) IOM sampler.
    C) Liquid sampler.
    D) Diffusion sampler.

6. Maintaining a constant flow rate during sampling is critical. Which of the following are devices that help maintain a constant flow during the sample period?

    A) Precision rotameter, laminar flow device.
    B) Flow rate meter, precision rotameter.
    C) Dry gas meter, wet gas meter.
    D) Pressure-compensating device, critical flow orifice.

7. There are two categories of calibration devices: primary and secondary. A primary device ____.

    A) Provides an indirect measurement of airflow.
    B) Includes a precision rotameter.
    C) Provides a direct measurement of airflow.
    D) Is independent of air pressure.

8. Sample breakthrough describes a condition where sampled material passes through the collection device and is captured on the back-up section. When the mass on the back-up exceeds ______, it means ________.

    A) 1%, the sample is invalid.
    B) Unity, the exposure exceeds safe levels.
    C) 10%, a significant portion of the contaminant may not have been collected.
    D) 5%, the front and back-up sections must be added to get a valid sample.

9. Why would a precision rotameter be placed in front of a sampling train during an exposure assessment?

    A) To verify the flow rate.
    B) To control the flow rate.
    C) To improve sample quality.
    D) To reduce continuous sample variability.

10. Using the lead extended work-shift formula: PEL ($\mu g/m^3$) = 400/hours worked in the day, what is the adjusted PEL for a 10-hour shift?

    A) 45 ug/m^3
    B) 42 ug/m^3
    C) 40 ug/m^3
    D) 33 ug/m^3

11. The internal column of a precision rotameter ______________ as the height of the rotameter increases.

    A) Decreases in diameter.
    B) Increases in diameter.
    C) Remains the same in diameter.
    D) Changes in material of construction.

12. The preferred analytical method for hexavalent chromium is OSHA ID 215. What is the sample media for this method?

    A) 37 mm 0.8 um MCE.
    B) 25 mm 0.8 um MCE.
    C) 37 mm 5um PVC.
    D) 25 mm 5um PVC.

13. A common liquid chemical in chiller units can poison the combustible gas sensors on some combustible gas detectors. Select the chemical that can poison the sensors:

    A) Silicone.
    B) Hydrogen peroxide.
    C) Argon.
    D) Ethyl-alcohol.

14. FIDs are good at detecting high concentrations of organic compounds (up to 50,000 ppm), but perform poorly at the sub-ppm range. Select the false statement about FIDs:

    A) The sensitivity increases as the number of carbon-hydrogen bonds in the compound increases.
    B) The sensitivity is lower for inorganic compounds.
    C) The sensitivity decreases as the number of carbon-hydrogen bonds in the compound increases.
    D) The sensitivity limits their usefulness in environments with many organic compounds.

15. Grab samples are best utilized for which of the following?

    A) Determining time weighted averages.
    B) Determining the concentration of a contaminant at a specific point in time.
    C) Determining compliance with an OSHA PEL.
    D) Calibrating equipment.

16. The sample flow rate for a pump was recorded as 1.7 L/m and a concentration of 100 mg/m^3 was determined based on the volume associated with the flow of 1.7 L/m. The flow rate was actually 2 L/m. What is the corrected concentration?

    A) 50 mg/m^3
    B) 85 mg/m^3
    C) 100 mg/m^3
    D) 117 mg/m^3

17. A 200 mL burette is being used to calibrate the flow rate of a pump. The soap bubble travels from zero to 200 mL in 19.8 seconds. Calculate the flow rate for the pump.

    A) 1000 mL/min
    B) 2.0 L/min
    C) 0.6 L/min
    D) 1000 cc/min

18. An air sample must be collected that can determine if exposures are less than 10% of the OEL. The literature shows the OEL is 10 mg/m^3. The lowest level of mass that can be detected by the analytical balance is 100 ug. The pump is calibrated at 2 L/min. What is the minimum amount of time that must be sampled to ensure the results will meet the desired goal of knowing the exposure can be as low as 10% of the OEL?

    A) 1 hour
    B) 20 min
    C) 30 min
    D) 50 min

19. To improve collection efficiency, two bubble samplers are placed in sequence in the sample train. If the collection efficiency for the target gas is 50%, what is the overall collection efficiency of the sample method?

    A) 100%
    B) 75%
    C) 66%
    D) 50%

20. All the following are methods for monitoring bioaerosols, except:

    A) An impactor with agar plates.
    B) Zefon Air-O-Cell cassettes.
    C) A 25-mm Cassette with non-conductive cowl.
    D) An Anderson-type (N6) single stage impactor.

Rubric 1: Air Sampling and Instrumentation Answers

1. Answer C.
   Explanation: Integrated air sampling involves the extraction of a gas or vapor from a sample airstream, followed by laboratory analysis. The two extraction techniques typically used include adsorption and absorption.
   Source: Fundamentals of Industrial Hygiene 6th ed. NSC

2. Answer A.
   Explanation: The formula used for sample volume:
   $$SV = \frac{LOD}{EL \times F}$$

   Where:
   SV is the minimum sample volume in liters
   LOD is the lower limit of detection in micrograms (ug)
   EL is the exposure limit in milligrams per cubic meter (mg/m^3)
   F is the expected percent of the exposure limit expressed as a decimal (.xx)

   Insert the known values and solve for SV:
   $$SV = \frac{10}{25\frac{mg}{m3} x.1}$$

   $$SV = 4\ L$$

   The formula for determining sample time (or volume or flow rate):
   $$T = \frac{SV}{FR}$$

   Where:
   T is time in minutes
   SV is the sample volume in liters
   FR is the flow rate in liters per minute

   Insert the known values and solve for T:
   $$T = \frac{4\ L}{0.1\ L/m}$$

   $$T = 40\ \text{minutes}$$

3. Answer B.
   Explanation: Most compliance sampling is *personal sampling*. The other answers are uses of *area sampling*.
   Source: Fundamentals of Industrial Hygiene 6th ed. NSC

---

4. Answer B.

    Explanation: Calculate and report fiber density on the filter, E (fibers/mm²), by dividing the average fiber count per graticule field, F/N_f, minus the mean field blank count per graticule field, B/N_b, by the graticule field area, A_f, (approx. 0.00785 mm²):

$$E_{fiber\ density} = \frac{\frac{F}{N_f} - \frac{B}{N_b}}{A_f}$$

Where:

$E_{fiber\ density}$ is the amount of fibers on the filter in fibers/mm²
f/N_f is the average or mean fiber count per graticule field
B/N_b is the mean fiber count per graticule field of the blank
A_f is the graticule field area (approximately 0.00785 mm²)

$$E_{fiber\ density} = \frac{3 - 0.01\ fibers}{0.00785\ mm^2}$$

$$E_{fiber\ density} = 381\ f/mm2$$

NOTE: Fiber counts above 1300 fibers/mm² and fiber counts from samples with >50% of filter area covered with particulate should be reported as "uncountable" or "probably biased." Other fiber counts outside the 100–1300 fiber/mm² range should be reported as having "greater than optimal variability" and as being "probably biased."
Source: NIOSH 7400

5. Answer D.

    Explanation: Diffusion or passive samplers allow personal sampling without an air pump.
    Source: Fundamentals of Industrial Hygiene 6th ed. NSC

6. Answer D.

    Explanation: Pressure compensating devices are designed to overcome flow rate variations due to filter loading or hose crimp. Critical flow orifice is a hole in a metal plate. The principle is to draw air through the orifice under critical-flow conditions and constant upstream pressure.
    Source: Fundamentals of Industrial Hygiene 6th ed. NSC

7. Answer C.

    Explanation: A secondary calibration device provides an indirect measure of airflow. An example of a secondary device is a precision rotameter.
    Source: Fundamentals of Industrial Hygiene 6th ed. NSC

8. Answer C.

    Explanation: If the mass on the back-up section exceeds 10% of the front section, then mass may not have been collected, and the results may not be valid.
    Source: Fundamentals of Industrial Hygiene 6th ed. NSC

9. Answer A.
   Explanation: If done as a brief check during sampling, the test can confirm the flow rate remains in the calibration range. Battery drain and filter loading are two conditions that can alter the pump flow rate.

10. Answer C.
    Explanation: PEL = 400/10   PEL = 40 ug/m^3
    Source: 29 CFR 1910.1025

11. Answer B.
    Explanation: Also known as variable area meters. They were invented by Karl Kuppers.

12. Answer C.
    Explanation: 37 mm 5um pore size PVC.

13. Answer A.
    Explanation: Other sensor poisons include sulfides and styrene.
    Source: The PID Handbook, Theory and Application of Direct Reading PID. Haag, W

14. Answer C.
    Explanation: FIDs are useful and sensitive to higher concentrations of single or known organic compounds with higher numbers of C-H bonds.
    Source: Fundamentals of Industrial Hygiene 6th ed. NSC

15. Answer B.
    Explanation: This makes grab samples useful for locating sources of exposure, screening for emergency response situations, and selection of PPE.

16. Answer B.
    Explanation: Determine the ratio of the flow rates 1.7/2 = 0.85, so 0.85 more air was drawn through the sample. Accordingly, the concentration is 0.85 less than the original. 0.85 x 100 mg/m^3 = 85 mg/m^3.

17. Answer C.
    Explanation:

$$200 \text{ mL}/19.8 \text{ sec} = 10.1 \text{ mL/sec}$$

$$\frac{10.1\ mL}{sec} \; x \; \frac{60\ sec}{min} \; x \; \frac{1\ L}{1000\ mL} = 0.6 \text{ L/min}$$

18. Answer D
    Explanation:
    Use the formula $\qquad$ t = m/QC
    Where:
    m = minimum detectable mass (mg)
    Q = sample flow (m3/min)
    C = threshold or minimum concentration to be measured (mg/m^3)

    Step 1: Convert detectable mass to mg.
    $$100 \text{ ug} \times \frac{1\,mg}{1000\,ug} = 0.1 \text{ mg}$$
    Step 2: Convert flow to m^3/min.
    $$\frac{2\,L}{min} \times \frac{1m^3}{1000\,L} = 0.002 \text{ m}^3/\text{min}$$

    Step 3: Determine minimum concentration.
    $$0.1 \times 10 \text{ mg/m}^3 = 1 \text{ mg/m}^3$$

    Step 4: Solve for t.
    $$t = m/QC$$

    $$t = 0.1 \text{ mg}/(0.002 \times 1 \text{ mg/m}^3)$$

    $$t = 50 \text{ min}$$

19. Answer: B
    Explanation: Bubble sampler one will capture 50% of the target gas and allow 50% to pass to bubble sampler two. Bubble sampler two will capture 50% of 50%, which is 25%. Accordingly, the overall efficiency is 75%.

20. Answer: C
    Explanation: The Anderson-type N6 is a single stage impactor that uses agar plates for viable samples and the Air-O-Cell cassettes are used for total fungal counts. The 25-mm cassette is utilized for fiber sampling and not used for fungal monitoring. *Source: ACGIH, Bioaerosols Assessment and Control*

Rubric 2: Analytical Chemistry

Analytical chemistry is the foundation of exposure monitoring for airborne contaminants. A valid analytical method must be utilized to obtain valid results.

This section focuses on the specific methods for determining the composition of substances. This discipline allows the practitioner to identify and quantify (numerical amount or concentration) the analyte. The analytical method utilized is based upon the analyte or contaminant in question.

When developing a sampling strategy, review the sampling and analytical methods available for the contaminants of interest. Numerous governmental and consensus organizations have compiled and published manuals of sampling and analytical methods. The most common are NIOSH and OSHA.

A general understanding of the analytical methods and procedures is important. This includes the following:

- Selecting the appropriate analyte and the analytical method.
- The requirements and limitations of the analytical method.
- Awareness of the possible interferences that may be present.

Once the sampling method is chosen and testing has concluded, the samples must be analyzed, and preferably by an accredited industrial hygiene laboratory. Laboratories conduct the specific analytical method depending on contaminant. Listed below are common analytical chemistry methods. *Source: The Occupational Environment- It's Evaluation, Control and Management- Chapter 12: Analysis of Gases and Vapors*

Gas Chromatography

Gas chromatography is a separation technique where components of a sample are separated by differential distribution between a gaseous mobile phase and a solid or liquid stationary phase held in a glass or metal column. A sample is injected into the carrier gas as a sharp plug and individual components are detected as they elute from the column at characteristic "retention times" after injection. *Source: Biological Monitoring Techniques for Human Exposure to Industrial Chemicals*

High Performance Liquid Chromatography

A chromatography process in which components of a mixture are separated in a two-phase system. In liquid chromatography (LC), the stationary phase consists of either a solid or a liquid that is coated on or bonded to a solid. The moving, or mobile, phase is a liquid. Conditions are established under which the individual components flow at different rates under the influence of the mobile phase. The differing rates of elution occur because of interaction between the sample components and the stationary phase.

There are four principal mechanisms in LC by which components of samples are selectively retained:

- Differences in partition coefficients (liquid-liquid chromatography)
- Differences in adsorption effects on surfaces such as silica gel (liquid-solid chromatography)
- Differences in dissociation of weak or strong electrolytes (ion-exchange chromatography)
- Differences in molecular size or shape (steric exclusion chromatography).

The mechanism resulting from differences in partition coefficients can be further subdivided into reversed-phase (RP) chromatography, in which hydrophobic interactions occur between the sample components and nonpolar groups. *Source: Biological Monitoring Techniques for Human Exposure to Industrial Chemicals*

Table 2.1: Summary of Liquid Chromatography Analytical Techniques Mass Spectroscopy

Analytical Technique	Type of Device	Selectivity (Application)	Examples of Common Analytes
Liquid Chromatography	HPLC: The analysis of nonvolatile organic compounds		
	Ion Chromatography: The analysis of acid vapors		
	Ultraviolet-Visible Detector	Aromatic organic compounds	acetaldehyde, anisidine, p-chlorophenol, diethylenetriamine, ethylenediamine, maleic anhydride, p-nitroaniline, polynuclear aromatics (PNAs) hexavalent chromium, ozone (Ion Chromatography)
	Fluorescence Detector	Aromatic Compounds	isocyanates, polynuclear aromatics, polynuclear aromatic hydrocarbons (PAHs)
	Electrochemical Detector	Aromatic Compounds Halogens	isocyanates and peroxides iodine, cyanides (Ion Chromatography)
	Conductivity Detector	Ionic species	aminoethanol compounds, ammonia, hydrogen sulfide, inorganic acids, iodine, hydrogen sulfide, sulfur dioxide

Mass spectroscopy yields detailed structural information about organic compounds and accurate elemental analysis of solid state samples. It is often possible to positively identify an unknown compound based on a detailed interpretation of the mass spectrum alone. The mass spectrometer produces charged particles from the sample molecules. These particles consist of a parent or molecular ion and ionic fragments of the original molecules. The ions are then sorted and detected according to their mass-to-charge ratio (m/e or m/z). The instrumentation required to generate the mass spectrum includes an inlet system for vaporization of the sample, an ionizing source where the sample is ionized, a mass analyzer which separates the ions according to their mass-to-charge ratio, and a detection system. See tables below of spectroscopy methods and applications. *Source: Biological Monitoring Techniques for Human Exposure to Industrial Chemicals*

Table: Summary of Spectroscopy Methods and Applications

Method	Selectivity (Application)	Example
Mass Spectroscopy	Identification of unknown organics	Indoor air, odor problems, byproduct identifications
Infrared Spectroscopy	Identification of unknown organics, screen wastes for disposal	Complementary analysis to confirm MS results, Oil mist in air
Visible and Ultraviolet Spectroscopy	Organic or inorganic compounds	Cr(VI), formaldehyde, ammonia
X-ray Powder Diffraction	Crystalline material	Silica and Chrysotile
X-ray Fluorescence	Elemental analysis	Lead

Table: Summary of Metal Analyses and Applications by Atomic Spectroscopy

Method	Selectivity (Application)	Example
Atomic Absorption- Flame	Metals, one metal at a time	Solder fumes
Graphite Furnace-Atomic Absorption	Trace metals	Arsenic Lead in drinking water
Cold Vapor Atomic Absorption	Specifically for mercury	Mercury
Hydride Atomic Absorption	Specifically for As & Se	Arsenic & Scandium
Inductively Coupled Plasma –Atomic Emission Spectroscopy	Simultaneous of sequential multi-metals analysis	Metal screening

IR Spectroscopy

Almost all substances, except monatomic and homopolar molecules (e.g., NE, HE, O_2, N_2), have absorption capacity in this region. No two compounds with different structures will have the same IR spectra. Limit of detection and sensitivity are low. Mixtures are difficult to analyze.
Source: Biological Monitoring Techniques for Human Exposure to Industrial Chemicals

Visible/UV Radiation

Electromagnetic radiation (visible and ultraviolet light) measures the wavelength and photons of energy. The absorption of UV causes energy changes involving the ionization of atoms and molecules. The type of spectrophotometer is either a prism or grate. The light (tungsten for visible and a hydrogen lamp for UV) is refracted into a spectrum. A series of slits limits the wavelength striking the sample. UV is very good for quantitative analysis, covers a wide range or organics and inorganics, and has high sensitivity. Limitations include temperature changes, ionization of solute and stray light. *Source: Biological Monitoring Techniques for Human Exposure to Industrial Chemicals*

Atomic Absorption Spectrophotometry

During the operation of an atomic absorption spectrophotometer, a spectrum of emission lines is radiated from the light source containing a cathode of the metal of interest and directed through the atomic vapor generated from the sample in a flame or another device. The metal of interest present in the ground atomic state absorbs the element-specific radiation from the light source. The monochromator isolates the resonance line selected for measurement and the detector/electronic system processes the signal output and records/displays the amount of analyte in the sample.

An atomic absorption spectrophotometer consists of four basic components:
- A modulated light source which generates an emission spectrum of the element of interest
- A mechanism by which a portion of the element of interest in the sample is converted to the ground atomic state
- A wavelength selector to isolate the resonance and non-absorbable lines in the spectrum
- A photodetector/electronic system

Source: Biological Monitoring Techniques for Human Exposure to Industrial Chemicals

Wet Chemical Methods

Wet chemical methods include qualitative chemical measurements, such as changes in color (colorimetry). and quantitative chemical measurements: gravimetry and titrimetry. Wet chemistry includes pH (acidity and alkalinity) testing. The most practiced wet chemical method used for industrial hygiene analyses is titration. Titration is a method or process of determining the concentration of a dissolved substance in terms of the smallest amount of reagent of known concentration required to bring about a given effect in reaction with a known volume of the test solution.
Source: Chemistry, The Central Science 11th edition

Microscopy

Phase-Contrast Microscopy (PCM). Light microscopy method used to analyze air samples for concentrations of asbestos in fibers per cubic centimeter of air sampled. Transmission Electron Microscopy (TEM): A method of analyzing and quantifying samples for the presence of asbestos. Unlike light microscopy, TEM can definitively distinguish between asbestos fibers and other types of fibers. TEM also has a far higher resolution than light microscopy methods.

Asbestos is routinely analyzed by size-selective microscopic counting. Optical (or electron) microscopy visualizes the collected fibers. The actual size of each particle determines if it gets measured. Under OSHA and the NIOSH "A" optical counting rules, the fiber must be >5 μm long and have an aspect ratio of at least 3:1. Under the more recent EPA electron microscope counting rules the fibers must be >0.5 μm long and meet a 5:1 aspect ratio. Neither of these procedures establishes an independent fiber diameter counting rule. *Source: Fundamentals of Industrial Hygiene 5th edition*

Laboratory Quality Assurance

Quality assurance needs to meet or exceed these categories:
- Data is scientifically valid
- Data is scientifically and legally defensible
- Accuracy of data is verified and precision of data is characterized.

The laboratory shall be accredited by a recognized national or international authority to determine the laboratory's capability to perform certain testing and measurement activities. AIHA Laboratory Accreditation Programs, LLC is a Full Member of the International Laboratory Accreditation Cooperation (ILAC) and a signatory (for testing) of the ILAC Mutual Recognition Arrangement (MRA). The program requires a laboratory to operate a management system that is compliant with ISO/ICE Standard 17025:2005, participate in interlaboratory proficiency demonstration programs, and meet other technical requirements. Biennially, the laboratory submits an application for review and is subjected to an on-site evaluation by a qualified individual. Laboratories that participate in this accreditation program have demonstrated an ability to perform industrial hygiene analyses. *Source: Industrial Hygiene Reference and Study Guide 3rd Edition*

Chain of Custody

This procedure tracks the history and control of samples received. The chain of custody includes the following: the date the sample was collected; the date the sample was shipped; the date the sample was received; the date the analyst received the sample; the date the analysis was completed; the date the analytical results were checked by another analyst; and the date the sample results were released by a supervisor or his/her representative. It is important to follow chain-of-custody requirements because it documents the proper handling of samples for litigation purposes. *Source: https://www.osha.gov/dts/osta/otm/otm_ii/otm_ii_1.html#appendix_II_11*

Definitions:

Accuracy- The agreement of a measured value to the accepted reference value.

Bias- The difference between a measured value and the true value.

Blank- Unexposed sample medium used to determine the quantity of analyte present in the media.

Breakthrough- Elution of the analyte of interest from the front section to the back section of a sorbent tube.

Calibration- The process determining the specific response of a device, such as an instrument, to a known value.

Desorption Efficiency- The fraction of collected analyte recovered from a sorbent tube.

Limit of Detection- The smallest quantity of analyte that can be distinguished from background noise by the instrument.

Matrix- The material sampled (e.g., air, water, soil, bulk substance).

Medium- The device or material used to collect the sample (e.g., filter, solid sorbent, impinger solution).

Precision- The reproducibility of individual measurements or variability.

Recovery- Fraction of analyte recovered from the sample medium during sample preparation and analysis.

Spike- A known quality of analyte added to the sampling medium for the purpose of determining desorption efficiency, determining recovery, or preparing quality control samples.

Equations:

BEER-LAMBERT LAW

$$\log \frac{I_0}{I} = abc$$

Where:

log I_0/I is the absorbance i.e. the spectrophotometer reading (A).

I_0 is the incident light beam intensity.

I is the exit light beam intensity.

a is the constant for molar absorptivity (L/g-cm).

b is the length of the path for the light beam (cm).

c is the concentration of material (g/L).

Use:

The basis of operation for the UV, Visible and IR spectrophotometry to determine the concentration of a contaminant in solution.

Example:

A solution of acetone in water is to be analyzed. The absorbance-concentration graph produces a straight line. If the molar absorptivity is 0.30 L/g-cm, the path length is 1 cm, and the absorbance is 0.400 at 265 nm, determine the concentration of the acetone.

$$\log \frac{I_0}{I} = abc$$

Step 1: Solve for the concentration-c

$$0.400 = 0.30 \text{ L/g-cm}(1 \text{ cm})(c)$$

$$\frac{0.400}{\left(0.30\frac{L}{g-cm}\right)(1 \ cm)} = c$$

$$1.33 \text{ g/L} = c$$

Source: Industrial-Occupational Hygiene Calculations: A Professional Reference

Rubric 2: Analytical Chemistry Questions

1. The partial pressures of a mixture of gasses are: 66% N_2, 10% O_2 and 24% CO_2 by volume at 1 atmosphere. What is the partial pressure of each gas in mmHg?

    A) $N_2 = 501.6$ mmHg, $O_2 = 76$ mmHg, and $CO_2 = 182.4$ mmHg.
    B) $N_2 = 0.66$ mmHg, $O_2 = 0.1$ mmHg, and $CO_2 = 0.24$ mmHg.
    C) $N_2 = 218$ mmHg, $O_2 = 218$ mmHg, and $CO_2 = 324$ mmHg.
    D) $N_2 = 253.3.6$ mmHg, $O_2 = 253.3$ mmHg, and $CO_2 = 1253.3$ mmHg.

2. X-ray fluorescence is a technique that analyzes the radiation emitted from the contaminant after exposure to x-rays. This technique is utilized for which of the following?

    A) Crystals in tissue analysis.
    B) Lead wipe sample analysis.
    C) Hydrocarbons in exhaled air.
    D) Halogens in urine.

3. The principle involved in neutron activation analysis consists of first irradiating a sample with neutrons in a nuclear reactor to produce specific radionuclides. Data reduction of __________ spectra then yields the concentrations of various elements in the samples being studied. With instrumental neutron activation analysis it is possible to measure quantitatively about 60 elements in small samples.

    A) X-ray.
    B) Gamma ray.
    C) Microwave.
    D) Infrared.

4. Given two spectrophotometer readings from two solutions, and the known equivalent molar concentrations, how is the molar concentration of an unknown solution determined from its spectrophotometer reading?

    A) Utilizing the principals of Fick's Law.
    B) Utilize the principals of Boyles Law.
    C) Utilize the principals of Bowes Law.
    D) Utilize the principals of Beers Law.

5. What is the appropriate method when sampling for Vinyl Chloride?

    A) NIOSH 1007.
    B) NIOSH 1200.
    C) NIOSH 1300.
    D) NIOSH 1301.

6. What is the duration of the AIHA Lab Accreditation?

   A) 1 year.
   B) 2 years.
   C) 3 years.
   D) 4 years.

7. When comparing the graphite furnace to the flame atomic absorption spectrophotometry, the primary advantage of the graphite furnace is:

   A) The analysis is more sensitive.
   B) The analysis is more specific.
   C) The analysis is easier to perform.
   D) The analysis is less accurate.

8. Which of the following is not true about the Beer-Lambert law?

   A) Relates the spectroscopic absorbance to the path-length of the sample cell.
   B) Uses the molar absorptivity as a constant of the proportionality.
   C) States the absorbance is inversely proportional to the analyte concentration.
   D) Correlates the observed spectroscopic absorbance of the concentration of the target analyte.

9. Select the analytical method that is most useful for the qualitative identification of an unknown organic compound.

   A) Gas chromatography
   B) Mass spectrophotometry
   C) High performance liquid chromatography
   D) Atomic Absorption Spectroscopy

10. Select the compound that is least likely to be quantitatively analyzed by infrared spectrophotometry.

    A) Benzo(a)pyrene on an XAD-2 tube.
    B) Oil mist on a PVC filter.
    C) Nitrous Oxide in a bag.
    D) Quartz (silica) on a PVC filter.

11. When conducting sampling for the alcohol Cyclohexanol, what is the recommended media?

    A) Solid Sorbent tube.
    B) 1 μm PTFE filter.
    C) 5 μm Pre-weighed PVC filter.
    D) Silica Gel Tube.

12. The most common method for analyzing metals is:

    A) Flame Ionization.
    B) Atomic Absorption.
    C) Electron Capture.
    D) Photoionization.

13. Which technique does not apply to sense a particular contaminant using a nondispersive infrared photometer?

    A) Selective frequency night source (laser).
    B) Selective filtering of the light source.
    C) Selective frequency detector.
    D) Selective frequency analyzer.

14. Choose the statement that best describes chromatography.

    A) A separation technique generally used for inorganic compounds. The separation allows the quantitation of several compounds in multiple analysis.
    B) A separation technique generally used for organic compounds. The separation allows the quantitation of several compounds in a single analysis.
    C) A technique used to analyze organic compounds.
    D) A separation technique that quantifies several compounds in multiple analysis.

15. Choose the characteristic that does not accurately describe a flame ionization detector (FID).

    A) Sensitive to most organic compounds.
    B) Exhibits a linear response over a wide dynamic range.
    C) Responds only to compounds that can be oxidized with carbon atoms.
    D) Most commonly used for ion chromatographic analysis of carbon containing compounds.

16. Choose the characteristic that does not accurately describe an electron capture detector (ECD).

    A) Pesticide and polychlorinated biphenyls (PCB) analysis.
    B) Analysis of non-chlorinated hydrocarbons.
    C) Analysis of fluorinated compounds, nitroaromatics, and PAHs.
    D) Selective to compounds that have an affinity for free electrons.

17. Mass spectrometry (MS) is used in conjunction with __________ to identify the component that is responsible for a specific GC peak.

    A) High performance liquid chromatography.
    B) Ion chromatography.
    C) Liquid chromatography.
    D) Gas chromatography.

18. Choose the statement that does not accurately describe high-performance liquid chromatography (HPLC).

    A) HPLC is a separation tool suitable for compounds that have high boiling points and low vapor pressures.

    B) HPLC is commonly used for PAHs and has been derived for airborne organics, such as isocyanates and aldehydes.

    C) HPLC uses liquid as the carrier of mobile phase.

    D) All of the above accurately describes HPLC.

19. A solution of methyl ethyl ketone in water is to be analyzed. The absorbance-concentration graph produces a straight line. If the molar absorptivity is 0.33 L/g-cm, the path length is 1 cm, and the absorbance is 0.400 at 265 nm, determine the concentration of the methyl ethyl ketone.

    A) mg/m^3

    B) 1.21 g/L

    C) 12 ppm

    D) 33 µg/L

20. Convert 65°F to Centigrade.

    A) 18.3

    B) 4.1

    C) 25

    D) 33

Rubric 2: Analytical Chemistry Answers

1. Answer A.
   Explanation:

   $$1 \text{ atm} = 760 \text{ mmHg} = P_{total}$$
   $$P_{total} = P(N_2) + P(O_2) + P(CO_2) = .66(760) + .1(760) + .24(760)$$

2. Answer B.
   Explanation: According to NIOSH publications, portable XRF can provide useful quantitative data for on-site risk assessment and clearance decisions for lead wipe samples. *Source: NIOSHTIC 20043982.*

3. Answer B.
   Explanation: After the irradiation, the characteristic gamma rays emitted by the decaying radionuclides are quantitatively measured by gamma spectroscopy, where the gamma rays detected at a particular energy are indicative of a specific radionuclide's presence. Also, x-rays do not originate in the nucleus. *Source: Cornell University, Ward Center for Nuclear Sciences.*

4. Answer D.
   Explanation: Absorbance *vs.* concentration is a linear relationship, therefore, use linear interpolation. Beers Law Absorbance $= \log \frac{I_0}{I}$

5. Answer A.
   Explanation: According to the NIOSH Manual of Analytical Methods, the appropriate method when sampling for Vinyl Chloride is NIOSH 1007 – solid sorbent tubes (2 – tandem) and analyzed by gas chromatography + FID. *Source: NIOSH Manual of Analytical Methods 4th edition*

6. Answer B.
   Explanation: The accreditation duration is 2 years per the AIHA Lab Accreditation Program LLC – module 3. This program has been in operation for more than 30 years.

7. Answer A.
   Explanation: The graphite furnace is more sensitive than AAS and is the most commonly used AA method. It is also more efficient. *Source: Modern Analytical Chemistry, D. Harvey, 2000.*

8. Answer C.
   Explanation: The **absorbance is proportional** to the analyte concentration. Beer-Lambert relates the absorbance to the path length of the sample cell, uses molar absorptivity as a constant of the proportionality, correlates the observed spectroscopic absorbance of the concentration of the target analyte and is useful for quantitative determination of the analyte concentration, but applies only to a restricted analyte concentration range. *Source: Rocky Mountain Center for Occupational and Environmental Health.*

9. Answer B.

    Explanation: The mass spectrophotometer is used for qualitative identification of organics and is located at the end of a gas chromatograph. It produces ions that are seen as peaks, which are called fragmentation patterns. *Source: Rocky Mountain Center for Occupational and Environmental Health.*

10. Answer A.

    Explanation: Benzo(a) pyrene is analyzed per NIOSH 5506 – HPLC fluorescence/UV. Oil mist on a PVC filter is analyzed per NIOSH 5206 – Infrared spectrophotometry. Nitrous Oxide in a bag is analyzed per NIOSH 6600 – Infrared spectrophotometry. Quartz (silica) on a PVC filter is analyzed per NIOSH 7603 – Infrared spectrophotometry. *Source: NIOSH Manual of Analytical Methods 4th edition*

11. Answer A.

    Explanation: According to the NIOSH Manual of Analytical Methods, method 1402, the recommended media when sampling for Cyclohexanol is a solid sorbent tube (coconut shell). The analysis is done via gas chromatography-FID. *Source: NIOSH Manual of Analytical Methods 4th edition*

12. Answer B.

    Explanation: Atomic absorption is an analytical technique which takes advantage of the characteristic absorption by metals of certain wavelengths of light. *Source: Applications and Computational Elements of Industrial Hygiene*

13. Answer D.

    Explanation: Selective frequency analyzer is not used to sense a particular contaminant using a nondispersive infrared photometer. Nondispersive means that the infrared light is not dispersed, and a grating serves to disperse the light source. A nondispersive infrared photometer can be used to selectively sense a particular contaminant by selective frequency night source (laser), selective filtering of the light source, and selective frequency detector.

14. Answer B.

    Explanation: Chromatography is a separation technique that is generally used for detection of organic compounds. The separation allows the quantitation of several compounds in a single analysis. The three types of chromatography are Gas Chromatography (GC), High Performance Liquid Chromatography (HPLC), and Ion Chromatography (IC). *Source: The Occupational Environment: Its Evaluation, Control and Management, 3rd edition & Applications and Computational Elements of Industrial Hygiene*

15. Answer D.

    Explanation: The detector most commonly used for gas chromatographic analysis of carbon containing compounds is a Flame Ionization Detector (FID). FIDs are non-specific and sensitive to most organic compounds, exhibit a linear response over a wide dynamic range, and respond only to compounds that can be oxidized with carbon atoms. *Source: Applications and Computational Elements of Industrial Hygiene*

16. Answer B.

   Explanation: The electron capture detector (ECD) is used for analysis of halogenated compounds at very low concentrations. Characteristics of EDs include pesticide and polychlorinated biphenyls (PCB) analysis, analysis of fluorinated compounds, nitroaromatics, and PAHs. EDs are selective to compounds that have an affinity for free electrons. Non-chlorinated hydrocarbons have little response. A disadvantage of (ECD) is its narrow range of linearity, which demands careful calibration in the range of interest. *Source: Applications and Computational Elements of Industrial Hygiene*

17. Answer D.

   Explanation: Mass spectrometry (MS) is used in conjunction with gas chromatography (GC) to identify the component that is responsible for a specific GC peak. The GC separates the mixture into components. The individual components are then analyzed by MS. MS fractures and ionizes the compounds, and then accelerates and separates them based on charge/mass ratio. *Source: Applications and Computational Elements of Industrial Hygiene*

18. Answer D.

   Explanation: High Performance Liquid Chromatography (HPLC) can be used for the analysis of any organic compound which can be dissolved. The following characteristics describe HPLC. HPLC is a separation tool suitable for compounds that have high boiling points and low vapor pressures. HPLC is commonly used for PAHs and have been derived for airborne organics, such as isocyanates and aldehydes. HPLC uses liquid as the carrier of mobile phase. *Source: Applications and Computational Elements of Industrial Hygiene*

19. Answer B.

   Explanation:

$$\log\frac{I_0}{I} = abc$$

$\log\frac{I_0}{I} = abc$ = absorbance

absorbance = 0.400

a = 0.33 L/g-cm

b = 1 cm

c = ?

Step 1: Solve for the concentration-c

$$0.400 = 0.33 \text{ L/g-cm}(1 \text{ cm})(c)$$

$$\frac{0.400}{\left(0.33\frac{L}{g-cm}\right)(1\ cm)} = c$$

$$1.21 \text{ g/L} = c$$

20. Answer A.

Explanation:

$$F = \frac{9}{5}C + 32$$

$$65 = \frac{9}{5}C + 32$$

$$(65 - 32)\frac{5}{9} = C$$

$$18.3 = C$$

Rubric 3: Basic Science

This section covers the areas of science that are important in the field of industrial or occupational hygiene. The subjects include chemistry, biochemistry, biology, anatomy, physiology, physics and mathematics.

Skin Anatomy and Physiology

The skin is the largest organ of the body with a surface area about $2m^2$ and is the first body barrier to make contact with a wide variety of industrial hazards. To cope with attack from heat, cold, moisture, radiation, bacteria, fungi and penetrating objects, the skin's tough, flexible layer provides protection from these hazards and provides countless processes that keep our body in proper working condition.

Occupational hazards make a worker's skin increasingly susceptible. Particular disorders that are visible in the skin do not arise in the skin but in other organs. This makes the skin an effective pre-warning system and is critical in physical diagnosis and identification of systemic diseases. A number of predisposing factors interrelate to determine the degree to which a person's skin responds to chemical, physical and biological efficacies. These include type of skin (pigmentation, dryness, amount of hair), age, sex, season, previous skin diseases, allergies and personal hygiene. Historical information indicates that dermatological conditions other than injuries are the second most common cause of all occupational diseases, accounting for 13 percent of all cases reported to the Bureau of Labor Statistics in previous years.

Even though occupational skin disorders are a significant cause of impairment and disability, most cases are preventable. By diagnosing early and accurately, these disorders can be quickly nullified before causing adverse health effects to humans and the environment.

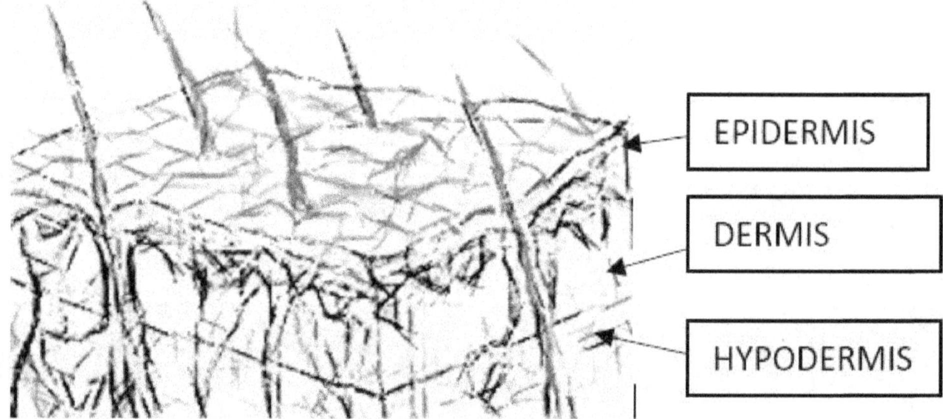

Important Terms and Concepts

Atopy- (uncommon or out of place) A relatively common genetic tendency toward the development of atopic dermatitis, asthma and hay fever.

Cutaneous- Pertaining to or affecting the skin.

Dermis- The deep fibrous, vascular inner layer of the skin. Second layer of the skin between the epidermis and the subcutaneous layer.

Dermatitis- Inflammation of the skin.

Dermatology- A branch of medicine concerned with the diagnosis, treatment (including surgery), and prevention of diseases of the skin, hair and nails.

Dermatosis- A broader term than dermatitis, including any cutaneous abnormality. Thus, it encompasses folliculitis, acne, pigmentary changes, nodules and tumors.

Epidermis- The outer layer of the skin. The top layer of the skin that is the thickest and contains melanocytes.

Gland- Any body organ that manufactures some liquid product and secretes it from its cells.

Hypodermis- Fat containing skin layer that insulates and provides a shock absorbing cushion.

Inflammation- The reaction of body tissue to injury by infection or trauma. The inflamed area is red, swollen, hot, and usually painful.

Keratin- Sulfur-containing proteins that form the chemical basis for epidermis tissues; found in nails, hair, and feathers.

Papillae- The top of the dermis made up of a layer of tiny cone- shaped objects.

Subcutaneous Layer- A layer of subcutaneous tissue with fatty and resilient elements that cushion and insulate the skin above it. Beneath the dermis.

Eye Anatomy and Physiology

The ability of the eye to translate radiant light energy into neural impulses, which are transmitted to the visual cortex of the brain, is highly important. Protection of the eye must be a priority in the field of health and safety.

The eye may absorb or be penetrated by hazardous substances. This is countered by covering or shielding the face and eye area. In one recent year, the Bureau of Labor Statistics reported 58,526 total cases of lost- time injuries or illnesses related to the eyes. The incidence rate was 6.6 per 10,000. These statistics represent only the OSHA- reportable injuries and illnesses.

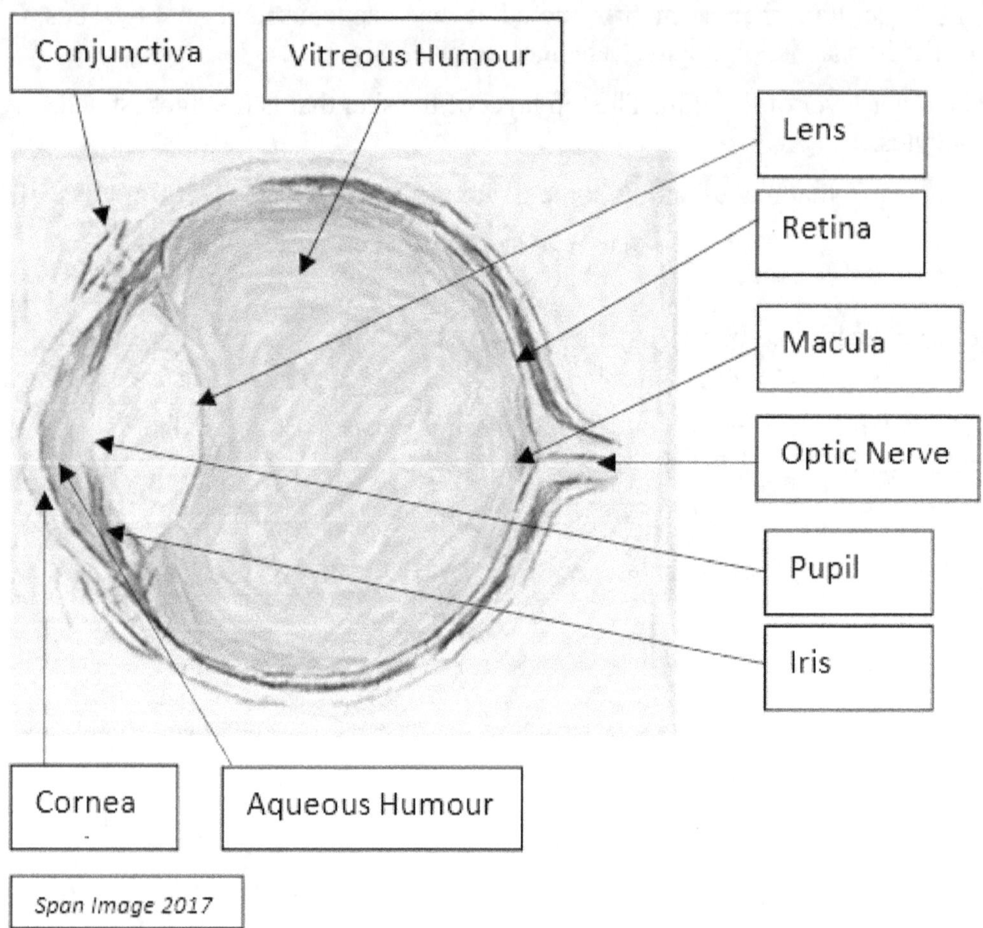

 Copyright©2019 SPAN International Training, LLC

Important Terms and Concepts

Astigmatism- A type of blurry vision caused by irregular curvature of the cornea.

Cataract- Opacity in the lens of the eye that may obscure vision.

Cornea- Transparent membrane covering the anterior portion of the eye.

Conjunctiva- The delicate mucous membrane that lines the eyelids and covers the exposed surface of the eyeball.

Conjunctivitis- Inflammation of the conjunctiva.

Emmetropia- A state of perfect vision.

Fovea- A depression or pit in the center of the macula of the eye; it is the area of clearest vision.

Keratitis- Inflammation of the cornea.

Nystagmus- Involuntary movement of the eyeballs.

Retina- The light-sensitive inner surface of the eye that receives and transmits images formed by the lens.

Pupil- The variable aperture in the iris through which light travels toward the interior regions of the eye. The pupil size varies from 2 mm to 8 mm.

Sclera- The tough white outer coat of the eyeball.

Vitreous humor- Jellylike fluid behind the lens of the eye.

Ear Anatomy and Physiology

The ear is made up of three parts: the outer, middle and inner ear. All the parts of the ear are important for detecting and transferring sound. The sense of hearing is based on the physics of sound and the physiology of the three parts of the ear, the nerves to the brain, and the brain regions involved in processing acoustic information.

Ear disorders can result in serious health consequences. Diagnosis of ear disorders are combated through the use of standardized audiometric testing. Damage to the ear can also result in multiple health concerns. Damage to the external and middle ear can cause conductive hearing loss. Dysfunction of the inner ear components consequents in sensorineural hearing loss and/or equilibrium problems. Ear damage and disorders can be mitigated by providing personal protective equipment and company enrollment in a hearing conservation program.

Source: Vander's Human Physiology- The Mechanism of Body Function

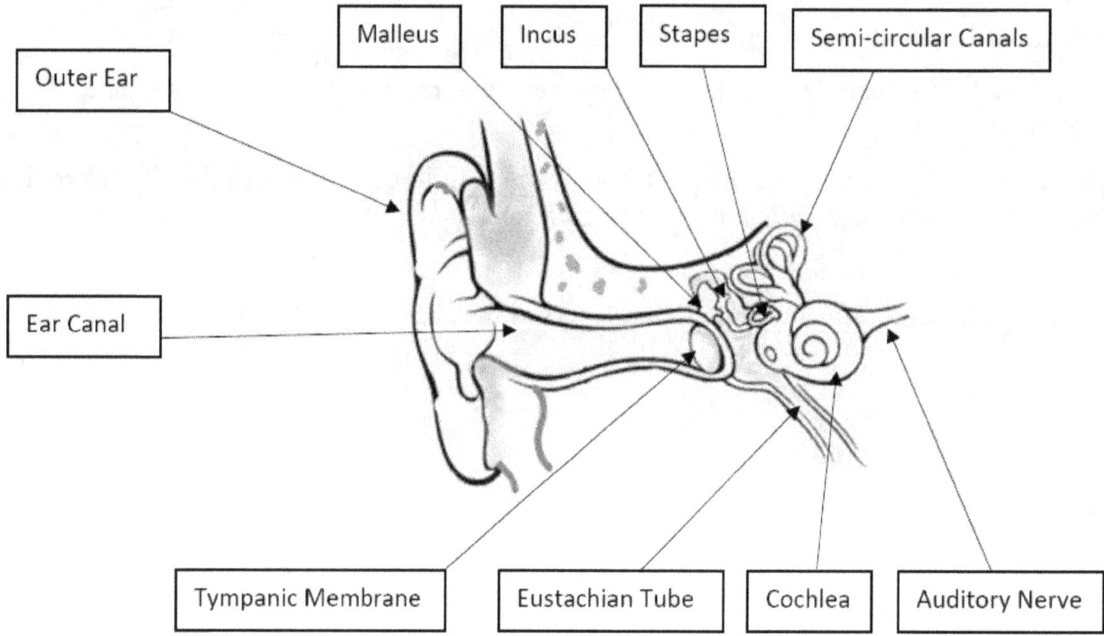

Important Terms and Concepts

Audiogram- A record of hearing loss or hearing level measured at several different frequencies—usually 500 to 6,000 Hz. The audiogram may be presented graphically or numerically. Hearing level is shown as a function of frequency.

Audible range- The frequency range across which normal ears hear: approximately 20 Hz to 20,000 Hz. Above the range of 20,000 Hz, the term *ultrasonic* is used. Below 20 Hz, the term *subsonic* is used.

Audible sound- Sound containing frequency components between 20 and 20,000 Hz.

Cerumen (Earwax) - Both sticky and bactericidal, cerumen prevents smaller particles from entering the ear canal and keeps the canal healthy and free of infection.

Cochlea- The auditory part of the internal ear shaped like a snail shell. It contains the basilar membrane on which the end organs of the auditory nerve are distributed.

Conductive hearing loss- Type of hearing loss not caused by noise exposure, but by any disorder in the middle or external ear that prevents sound from reaching the inner ear.

Eustachian tube- A structure about 2.5 in. (6 cm) long leading from the back of the nasal cavity to the middle ear. It equalizes the pressure of air in the middle ear with that outside the eardrum.

External auditory canal- The external auditory canal (meatus) is a skin-lined pouch about 1.5 in. (3.8 cm) long, supported in its outer third by the cartilage of the auricle and in its inner two-thirds by the bone of the skull. The cartilaginous meatus is curved and lies at an angle to the bony part, thus protecting the tympanic membrane and middle ear lying beyond it from direct trauma.

External ear- The external ear is composed of the auricle, or pinna, and the external auditory canal.

Frequency (in Hz)- Rate at which pressure oscillations are produced. One hertz is equivalent to one cycle per second. A subjective characteristic of sound related to frequency is pitch.

Hearing conservation- The prevention or minimizing of noise-induced deafness through the use of hearing protection devices, the control of noise through engineering methods, annual audiometric tests, and employee training.

Hearing level- The deviation in decibels of an individual's threshold from the zero reference of the audiometer.

Nosoacusis- Hearing losses due to diseases such as mumps; rubella; Meniere's disease; ototoxic drugs and chemicals; barotrauma; and trauma to the head.

Ossicle- Any member of a chain of three small bones from the outer membrane of the tympanum (eardrum) to the membrane covering the oval window of the inner ear.

Pinna- Ear flap; the part of the ear that projects from the head. Also known as the auricle.

Presbycusis- Hearing loss caused by age.

Sensorineural- Type of hearing loss that affects millions of people. If the inner ear is damaged, the hearing loss is sensory; if the fibers of the eighth nerve are affected, it is a neural hearing loss. Because the pattern of hearing loss is the same in either case, the term sensorineural is used.

Sound level- A weighted sound-pressure level obtained by the use of metering characteristics and the weighting A, B, or C specified in ANSI S1.4.

Temporary threshold shift (TTS) - The hearing loss suffered as the result of noise exposure, all or part of which is recovered during an arbitrary period of time when one is removed from the noise. It accounts for the necessity of checking hearing acuity at least 16 hours after a noise exposure.

Tinnitus- A perception of sound arising in the head. Most often perceived as a ringing or hissing sound in the ears. Can be the result of high frequency hearing loss.

Respiratory System Anatomy and Physiology

The respiratory system is vital for the human body to function. It consists of all the organs of the body that contribute to normal respiration of breathing, including all air passages: nose, mouth, upper throat, larynx, trachea and bronchi. The lungs are the location of oxygen transfer to the blood and carbon dioxide removal from the blood. Finally, the diaphragm and the muscles of the chest perform normal respiratory movements.

Human cells obtain most of their energy from chemical reactions involving oxygen. The main process is metabolism. During this process, each cell consumes oxygen and produces carbon dioxide as a waste substance.

Anything affecting the respiratory system, whether it is insufficient oxygen or contaminated air, can affect the entire human organism. This system is a direct avenue of entry for toxic materials. This is because of its direct association with the circulatory system and the ongoing need to oxygenate human tissue cells.

Important Terms and Concepts

Alveoli- Tiny air sacs of the lungs, formed at the ends of bronchioles; through the thin walls of the alveoli, the blood takes in oxygen and gives up carbon dioxide in respiration.

Bronchiole- The slenderest of the many tubes that carry air into and out of the lungs.

Bronchitis- Inflammation of the bronchi or bronchial tubes.

Cilia- Tiny hair-like whips in the bronchi and other respiratory passages that aid in the removal of dust trapped on these moist surfaces.

Emphysema- A lung disease in which the walls of the air sacs (alveoli) have been stretched too thin and have broken down.

Esophagus- The part of the alimentary canal that connects the throat to the stomach: the gullet. In humans and other vertebrates, it is a muscular tube lined with mucous membrane.

Inspiration- The movement of air from the external environment through the airways into the alveoli during breathing.

Larynx- The organ by which the voice is produced. It is situated at the upper part of the trachea.

Metabolism- The process through which the body combines oxygen with food substances, and thus produces energy.

Mucociliary Escalator- In addition to the mucus, the membrane is coated with cilia, or hair-like filaments, that move in coordinated waves to propel mucus and trapped particles toward the nostrils. The mucociliary escalator is a major barrier against infection and minimizes pulmonary particle deposition.

Nasal septum- A narrow partition that divides the nose into right and left nasal cavities.

Nasopharynx- Upper extension of the throat.

Pharynx- A tubular passageway attached to the base of the skull and extending downward behind the nasal cavity, the mouth, and the larynx to continue to the esophagus.

Pleura- The thin membrane investing the lungs and lining the thoracic cavity, completely enclosing a potential space known as the pleural cavity.

Pleurisy- Caused when the outer lung lining (visceral pleura) and the chest cavity's inner lining (parietal pleura) lose their lubricating properties; the resultant friction causes irritation and pain.

Pneumoconiosis- Literally "dusty lungs;" a result of the continued inhalation of various kinds of dust or other particulates; the tissue reaction resulting from the accumulation of such dusts in the lungs.

Pneumonitis- Inflammation of the lungs.

Respiration (primary meaning) - The tissue enzyme oxidation processes that use oxygen and produce carbon dioxide. More generally, this term designates the phases of oxygen supply and carbon dioxide removal.

Respiration (secondary meaning) - The enzymatic processes in the tissues that use oxygen and produce carbon dioxide. The blood contains a chemical that is part protein and part iron pigment, called hemoglobin. The hemoglobin binds oxygen when the blood flows through regions where oxygen is plentiful—as in the alveoli—and releases it to tissues that are consuming oxygen.

Rhinitis- Inflammation of the mucous membrane lining in the nasal passages.

Thoracic and alveolar deposition- The respiratory tract is a highly efficient dust collector. All particles entering the respiratory system larger than 4 or 5 micrometers (µm) are deposited in it. Half of those of 1-µm size appear to be deposited and the other half exhaled. The sites of deposition in the system are different for various sizes. Particles greater than 2.5 or 3 µm equivalent size are deposited in the upper respiratory system. Particles 2 µm in equivalent size are deposited about equally in the upper respiratory system and in the alveolar or pulmonary air spaces. Particles about 1 µm in equivalent size are deposited more efficiently in the alveolar spaces.

Trachea- The windpipe, or tube that conducts air to and from the lungs. It extends between the larynx above and the point where it divides into two bronchi below.

Turbinates- A series of scroll-like bones in the nasal cavity that serves to increase the amount of tissue surface exposed in the nose, permitting incoming air to be moistened and warmed prior to reaching the lungs (also known as conchae).

General Sciences

This section includes chemistry, physics and mathematics as they apply to the industrial – occupational health and hygiene profession.

Important Terms and Concepts

Acid – A substance that is able to donate a proton and thereby increase the concentration of H^+(aq) when dissolved in water.

Atom – The smallest representative particle of an element.

Atomic Weight – The average mass of the atoms of an element. It is numerically equal to the mass in grams of one mole of the element.

Base – A substance that is an H^+ acceptor and produces an increase of OH^- (aq) when dissolved in water.

Combustible – Capable of catching fire or burning.

Combustible liquids – Combustible liquids are those having a flash point at or above 100 °F (37.8°C).

Flammable – The capability of a substance to be set on fire or support combustion easily.

Flammable Liquid – Any liquid having a flash point below 100 °F (37.8°C).

Flash Point – The lowest temperature at which a liquid gives off enough vapor to form an ignitable mixture with air and produce a flame when a source of ignition is present. Two tests are used: open cup and closed cup.

Free Radical – A substance with 1 or more unpaired electrons.

Isomers – Substances with the same composition but different structure.

NTP (normal temperature and pressure) – A gas industry reference base. May vary from country to country. Normal, or ambient temperature is 70°F (21°C). Normal pressure is one atmosphere (760 mmHg).

Poise (symbol: P) – Poise is the "cgs" unit of viscosity. Poise is equivalent to dyne-second per square centimeter. Poise is defined as the viscosity of a fluid in which a tangential force of 1 dyne per square centimeter maintains a difference in velocity of 1 centimeter per second between two parallel planes 1 centimeter apart. For high viscosity fluids, the common unit is centipoise (cP). Centipoise (cP) is 0.01 poise.

- CGS unit = centimeter-gram-second system of units.

- Dyne = a unit of force that, acting on a mass of one (1) gram, increases its velocity by one centimeter per second along the direction that it acts.

- Dyne-second per square centimeter (dyn x s/cm^2) is a non-SI measurement unit of dynamic viscosity in the centimeter-gram-second (CGS) system of units. It is equivalent to the CGS base viscosity unit named poise (P).

Reactive – Chemical reaction with the release of energy. Undesirable effects (e.g., pressure build up, temperature increase, formation of noxious, toxic, or corrosive byproducts) may occur because of the reactivity of a substance to heating, burning, direct contact with other materials, or other conditions in use of in storage.

STP (standard temperature and pressure) – STP is commonly used to define standard conditions for temperature and pressure, which is important for the measurements and documentation of chemical and physical processes - *0^oC (273.1^oK, 32^oF) and 1 atm.*

Volatile – Tendency to evaporate.

Metric Unit Table

Prefix	Symbol	Value	Example
tetra	T	$1{,}000{,}000{,}000{,}000 = 10^{12}$	1 tetrameter (Tm) = 10^{12} m
giga	G	$1{,}000{,}000{,}000 = 10^9$	1 gigameter (Gm) = 10^9 m
mega	M	$1{,}000{,}000 = 10^6$	1 megameter (Mm) = 10^6 m
kilo	k	$1{,}000 = 10^3$	1 kilogram (kg) = 10^3 g
hecto	h	$100 = 10^2$	1 hectogram (hg) = 100 g
deka	da	$10 = 10^1$	1 dekaliter (daL) = 10 L
deci	d	$0.1 = 10^{-1}$	1 deciliter (dL) = 0.1 L
centi	c	$0.01 = 10^{-2}$	1 centimeter (cm) = 0.01 cm
milli	m	$0.001 = 10^{-3}$	1 milligram (mg) = 0.001 g
micro	μ	$0.000\ 001 = 10^{-6}$	1 micrometer (μm) = 10^{-6} m
nano	n	$0.000\ 000\ 001 = 10^{-9}$	1 nanogram (ng) = 10^{-9} g
pico	p	$0.000\ 000\ 000\ 001 = 10^{-12}$	1 picogram (pg) = 10^{-12} g
femto	f	$0.000\ 000\ 000\ 000\ 001 = 10^{-15}$	1 femtogram = 10^{-15} g

Vapor Hazard Ratio

$$Vapor\ Hazard\ Ratio = \frac{saturation\ concentration}{exposure\ guideline}$$

Where:
Vapor/Hazard Ratio is an indicator of relative risk (unitless).
Saturation concentration is the saturation or equilibrium concentration of a gas or vapor (parts per million) at NTP.
Exposure guideline is an exposure limit, such as TLV, PEL, MAK (parts per million).

Use:
Calculating the relative risk aids in assigning respiratory protection, allows for comparison of vapor based hazards between chemicals (exposure and even flammability).
Note: Higher ratios indicate the hazard is more likely in the vapor phase rather than saturation phase.

Example:
What is the vapor hazard ratio for methylene chloride, and does the hazard exist in vapor form or saturation form first? Literature states the saturation concentration is 550,000 parts per million. OSHA defines the permissible exposure limit as 25 parts per million.

Step 1: Calculate the vapor/hazard ratio

$$Vapor\ Hazard\ Ratio = \frac{saturation\ concentration}{exposure\ guideline}$$

$$Vapor\ Hazard\ Ratio = \frac{550,000\ ppm}{25\ ppm}$$

$$Vapor\ Hazard\ Ratio = 22,000$$

The ratio is much higher than the exposure limit; therefore, the hazard most likely occurs in the vapor form before saturation.

Parts Per Million: Volume/Volume

$$ppm = \frac{V_{cont}}{V_{air}} \; x \; 10^6$$

Where:
V_{cont} is the volume of the contaminant in any volume unit (liters, cubic meters, cubic feet).
V_{air} is the volume of the space (room, tedlar bag) in any volume unit (liters, cubic meters, cubic feet). Units for both Vs must be the same.
ppm is parts per million.

Use:
To calculate the airborne concentration of a gas or vapor in parts per million based in the vapor volume of the contaminants and the volume of the space. The formula can be used to estimate the airborne exposure levels or calibration standard concentrations.

Example:
One pound-mole of toluene is spilled into a room that is 100 feet by 20 feet by 10 feet. The temperature in the room is approximately 75^0 F. Atmospheric pressure is estimated at 760 mmHg. Calculate the concentration in parts per million.

The conditions are similar to NTP. The volume that one pound-mole will occupy is 387 ft^3. The room volume is 20000 ft^3. Based on this information, calculate the volume/volume concentration.

$$ppm = \frac{V_{cont}}{V_{air}} \; x \; 10^6$$

$$ppm = \frac{387 \; ft^3}{20000 \; ft^3} \; x \; 10^6$$

$$ppm = 19{,}350 \; ppm$$

This is the theoretical maximum concentration, assuming the equilibrium or saturation has not been reached. This level is above IDLH of 2000 ppm and above the LEL of 1.1% (11,000 ppm).

Parts Per Million: Pressure/Pressure

$$ppm = \frac{P_v}{P_{atm}} \; x \; 10^6$$

Where:

P_v is the vapor pressure of the contaminant at a given temperature (mmHg).

P_{atm} is the atmospheric pressure (mmHg).

Note: 10^6 is the factor to convert the value to parts per million (ppm).

Use:

To calculate the maximum possible concentration of a gas or vapor in parts per million based on a pressure to pressure relationship. This is the saturation or equilibrium concentration – based on an environment with static conditions.

Note: This value may be less than the calculated volume/volume concentration because the entire volume of contaminant may not evaporate due to saturation.

Example:

Calculate the saturation concentration for acetone for the following conditions. The temperature is 70^0F and the barometric pressure is 1 atmosphere. The safety data sheet lists the vapor pressure of acetone at this temperature is 181 mmHg.

Step 1: Convert 1 atmosphere to mmHg
1 atm = 760 mmHg

Step 2: Calculate the concentration in ppm

$$ppm = \frac{P_v}{P_{atm}} \; x \; 10^6$$

$$ppm = \frac{181}{760} \; x \; 10^6$$

$$ppm = 238158$$

Converting from PPM to mg/M³

$$ppm = \frac{mg/m^3 \times 24.45}{MW}$$

Where:
PPM is the concentration in parts per million (volume/volume).
MG/M³ is the concentration in milligrams per cubic meter (mass/volume).
MW is the molecular weight of the element.
24.45 is the molar volume of air in liters at NTP conditions.

Use:
Allows for conversion between concentrations forms for problem solving.

Example:
Convert 100 ppm of toluene to mg/m³. Your reference material lists the Molecular weight of toluene as 92.

$$ppm = \frac{mg/m^3 x 24.45}{MW}$$

$$100\ ppm = \frac{mg/m^3 x 24.45}{92}$$

$$92\ x100 = mg/m^3 \ x\ 24.45$$

$$mg/m^3 = \frac{92\ x\ 100}{24.45}$$

$$= 376\ mg/m^3$$

The General Gas Law

$$\frac{P_1 V_1}{nRT_1} = \frac{P_2 V_2}{nRT_2}$$

Where:
n is the amount of moles of gas or vapor (unitless).
T is the absolute temperature in Kelvin (K) or Rankine (°R).
V_1 and V_2 are the vapor or gas volumes for conditions 1 and 2 (Liters).
R is the constant. See formula: $\left(\dfrac{0.082\ liters\ atmospheres}{moles\ K}\right)$
P_1 and P_2 are the vapor or gas pressures for conditions 1 and 2 (mm Hg).

Use:
To adjust the volume of a gas-air or vapor-air mixture when temperature AND pressure changes occur. Allows for prediction of effects on gas or vapor when ambient conditions change.

NOTE: The temperature must be in absolute units. Since n and R are constants, they can be dropped from both sides of the equation.

Example:
How many liters does one (1) gram-mole of hydrogen sulfide gas occupy at 20°C and 740 mm Hg?

Given: Gram-mole of H_2S @ 20°C and 740 mm Hg.

Step 1: Calculate volume occupied

Use: Combined Gas Law

$$\frac{P_1 V_1}{T_1} = \frac{P_2 V_2}{T_2}$$

Known: STD Conditions:
P_1 = 760 mm Hg
V_1 = 22.4 liters
T_1 = 273°K
P_2 = 740 mm Hg
V_2 = ?
T_2 = 293°K

Solving for V_2

$$V_2 = \frac{P_1 V_1 T_2}{P_2 T_1} = \frac{(760\ mm\ Hg)(22.4\ liters)(293°K)}{(740\ mm\ Hg)(273°K)}$$

$$V_2 = 24.7\ liters$$

OR

$$(22.4\ liters)\left(\frac{760\ mm\ Hg}{740\ mm\ Hg}\right)\left(\frac{293°K}{273°K}\right) = 24.7\ liters$$

Dalton's Law & Raoult's Law

$$P_{total} = X_1 P_1 + X_2 P_2 + \cdots + X_i P_i$$

Where:

P_{total} is the total pressure (mmHg).

$P_{1\ldots I}$ is the partial pressure of the specific gas (mmHg).

$X_{1\ldots I}$ is the mole fraction of the specific gas (unitless).

Use:

Calculate total pressures for gasses (Dalton) or liquid vapors (Raoult) in a mixture, which can then be used in airborne concentration modeling.

Example:

A gaseous mixture made from 6.00 g O_2 and 9.00 g CH_4 is placed in a 15.0-L vessel at 0°C. What is the partial pressure of each gas, and what is the total pressure in the vessel in mm Hg?

Note: Since each gas behaves independently, we can use the ideal-gas equation to calculate the pressure that each would exert if the other were not present. The total pressure is the sum of these two partial pressures.

Step 1: Convert the mass of each gas to moles

$$n_{O_2} = (6.00 \; g \; O_2)\left(\frac{1 \; mol \; O_2}{32.0 \; g \; O_2}\right) = 0.188 \; mol \; O_2$$

$$n_{CH_4} = (9.00 \; g \; CH_4)\left(\frac{1 \; mol \; CH_4}{16.0 \; g \; CH_4}\right) = 0.563 \; mol \; CH_4$$

Step 2: Use ideal-gas equation to calculate the partial pressure of each gas

$$P_{O_2} = \frac{n_{O_2}RT}{V} = \frac{(0.188 \; mol)(\frac{0.082 \; liters \; atmosphere}{moles \; k})(273 \; K)}{15.0 \; L} = 0.281 \; atm$$

$$P_{CH_4} = n_{CH_4}RT = \frac{(0.563 \; mol)\left(\frac{0.082 \; liters \; atmosphere}{moles \; k}\right)(273 \; K)}{15.0 \; L} = 0.841 \; atm$$

Step 3: Use Dalton's Law to calculate the total pressure in the vessel

$$P_T = P_{O_2} + P_{CH_4} = 0.281 \; atm + 0.841 \; atm = 1.122 \; atm$$

Step 4: Convert from atm to mm Hg

$$(1.122 \; atm)\left(\frac{760 \; mm \; Hg}{1 \; atm}\right) = 852.7 \; mm \; Hg$$

Source: Chemistry- The Central Science (11th edition)

Reynold's Number Particulate

$$R_e = \frac{\rho d v}{\eta}$$

Where:

R_e is a dimensionless number that represents fluid flow around a particle.

η is the viscosity of the gas (air) in Poise. Poise = 1 g/cm-s in the old cgs units.

ρ is the density of the gas (air).

υ is the relative velocity of gas or particle (cm/sec).

d is the diameter of the particle (centimeters).

Use:

Calculation used to characterize the level of turbulence of air flow around a particle. Can either be gas flow around a particle or the around a particle or the settling of a particle through a gas.

NOTE: If CGS units at 20^0C the formula simplifies to:

$$R_e = Vd$$

The aerosols' Reynolds number (Re_p) is a dimensionless parameter to characterize fluid flow around an object. It is the ratio of inertial forces to viscous forces acting on the aerosol. By definition, when R_e is greater than 1000, the flow is turbulent. If the R_e is less than 1, the flow is laminar. If R_e is between 1 and 1000, then the flow is in the transition regime.

Example:

Calculate the Reynold's number for a mineral oil droplet (3 μm diameter) settling in calm air. The settling velocity is 0.04 cm/sec. The density of air is 1.205×10^{-3} g/cm^3 and the viscosity is 1.81×10^{-4} Poise.

Step 1: Convert diameter to cm

$$3 \text{ μm} = 0.0003 \text{ cm}$$

Step 2: Solve for R_e

$$R_e = \frac{\rho d v}{\eta}$$

$$R_e = \frac{1.205 \times 10^{-3} \frac{g}{cm^3}(0.0003 \; cm)(0.04 \frac{cm}{sec})}{1.81 \times 10^{-4}}$$

$$= 7.9 \times 10^{-5}$$

Accordingly, the R_e is much less than 1 and the flow is considered laminar.

Terminal Settling Velocity

$$V_{TS} = \frac{g d_p^2 (\rho_\rho - \rho_\alpha)}{18\eta}$$

Where:
V_{TS} is the terminal settling velocity (cm/sec).
g is acceleration due to gravity (cm/sec^2).
d_p is the particle diameter (cm).
ρ_p is the particle density (g/cm^3).
ρ_α is the air density (g/cm^3).
η is the air viscosity (Poise).

Use:
To calculate theoretical time required for particles to fall out of air. Some air pollution, filters, and sampling devices utilize this concept.

Note: Extremely small particles require an additional correction factor.

Example:
A battery manufacturing plant dumps lead oxide into a hopper. The mean lead oxide particle diameter is 3.5 μm. The hopper is located inside a closed room with no ventilation. The density of lead oxide is 9.53 g/cm^3. The gravitational force is 981 cm/sec^2. The temperature in the room is approximately 75°F. Literature indicates that the density of air is 1.2 x 10^{-3} g/cm^3 with a viscosity of 1.81 x 10^{-4} Poise. Calculate the terminal settling velocity for lead oxide particles that have become airborne in this room.

Step 1: Convert the diameter to cm

$$3.5 \ \mu m = 0.00035 \ cm$$

Step 2: Solve for V_{TS}

$$V_{TS} = \frac{g d_p^2 (\rho_\rho - \rho_\alpha)}{18\eta}$$

$$V_{TS} = \frac{981 \frac{cm}{sec^2} x (0.00035 \ cm)^2 x (9.53 - 1.2 \ x 10^{-3}) g/cm^2}{18(1.81 x 10^{-4} \ Poise)}$$

$$V_{TS} = 0.35 \ cm/sec$$

pH Calculation

$$pH = -log[H^+]$$

Where:
pH is the descriptor of acidity or alkalinity of a liquid (range 0 - 14 with no units).
log is the base 10 logarithm.
H^+ is the hydrogen ion concentration (molar: moles per liter).

Use:
To calculate pH or concentration of hydrogen ions.

Note: 7 is neutral while less than 7 is acid and greater than seven is alkaline.

Example:
Calculate the pH of 0.2 M hydrochloric acid. Molar is moles of solute per liter of solution.

Step 1: Solve for the concentration of H^+ ions

$$HCl \rightarrow H^+ + Cl^-$$

Since the relationship above is 1 to 1, 1 mole of HCl ionizes to 1 mole of H^+ ions, then 0.2 moles of HCL will ionize to 0.2 moles of H^+ ions.

Step 2: Solve for pH

$$pH = -log[H^+]$$

$$pH = -log[0.2]$$

$$pH = 0.69$$

Example:
Calculate the pH of a basic solution with an [OH⁻] value of 2.0 x 10⁻³.

Step 1: Calculate the [H⁻] value

$$[H^+] = \frac{K_w}{[OH^-]}$$

Note: K_w is the ion-product constant for water; 1 x 10⁻¹⁴ at 25⁰C.

$$[H^+] = \frac{1.0\ x\ 10^{-14}}{2.0\ x\ 10^{-3}}$$

$$H^= = 5 \text{ x } 10^{-12} \text{ M}$$

Step 2: Solve for pH

$$pH = -log[H^+]$$

$$pH = -log[5x10^{-12}]$$

$$pH = 11.3$$

Source: Chemistry, The Central Science 11ᵗʰ ed.

Acid Dissociation Constant

$$K_a = \frac{[H^+] x [A^-]}{[HA]}$$

Where:
K_a is the acid dissociation constant (no units).
$[H^+]$ is the hydrogen ion concentration (molar).
$[A^-]$ is the anion or conjugate base concentration (molar).
HA is the original acid concentration (molar).

Use:
To calculate the strength of an acid. A value of 1 is the maximum and represents a very strong acid.

Example:
Calculate the dissociation constant for 0.1 M acetic acid (CH_3COOH). The acid has a hydrogen ion concentration of 1.32×10^{-3} M.

Step 1: Write the reaction

$$CH_3COOH \rightarrow CH3COO^- + H^+$$

Step 2: Generate an ICE table (Initial, Change, & Equilibrium conditions)

	CH_3COOH	$CH3COO^-$	H^+
I	0.1 M	0	0
C	-1.32×10^{-3}	1.32×10^{-3}	1.32×10^{-3}
E	0.09868 M	1.32×10^{-3}	1.32×10^{-3}

Note: C is a 1 to 1 to 1 reaction, therefore if H^+ increases, then the CH_3COOH decreases. Total each column for Equilibrium.

Step 3: Solve for the dissociation constant (K_a)

$$K_a = \frac{[H^+] x [A^-]}{[HA]}$$

$$K_a = \frac{[1.32 x 10^{-3}] x [1.32 x 10^{-3}]}{[0.09868]}$$

$$K_a = 1.77 \times 10^{-5}$$

Since K_a is much smaller than 1, it is a weak acid.
Source: Chemistry, The Central Science 11th edition

Base Dissociation Constant

$$K_b = \frac{[BH^+][OH^-]}{B}$$

Where:
K_b is the base dissociation constant (no units).
OH^- is the concentration of the hydroxide ion (molar).
BH^+ is the concentration of the positive ion (molar).
B is the concentration of the base reagent (molar).

Use:
To calculate the strength of a base. A large value represents a strong base.

Example:
Calculate the base dissociation constant for an ammonia and water solution. The pH was measured at 10.5 and the equilibrium constant for ammonia is 0.00056 M.

Step 1: Write the reaction

$$NH_3 + H_2O \rightarrow NH_4^+ + OH^-$$

Step 2: Solve for pOH

Given that pH + pOH = 14, then

$$pOH = 14 - pH$$

$$pOH = 14 - 10.5 = 3.5$$

Step 3: Solve for OH^-

$$pOH = -\log[OH^-]$$

$$3.5 = -\log[OH^-]$$

$$-3.5 = \log[OH^-]$$

$$[OH^-] = 10^{-3.5}$$

$$= 0.0003 \text{ M}$$

Note: There is a 1 to 1 to 1 relationship in the dissociation reaction

Step 4: Solve for the base dissociation constant

$$K_b = \frac{[0.0003][0.0003]}{0.00056}$$

$$= 1.6 \times 10^{-4}$$

Source: Chemistry - The Central Science 11th edition

The following table lists H^+ concentrations and pH values of some common substances at 25°C. The pH of a solution can be estimated using the benchmark concentrations of H^+ and OH^- corresponding to whole number pH values.

Table: Relationship of H^+ concentrations and pH

	$[H^+]$ (M)	pH	pOH	$[OH^-]$ (M)
	$1\ (1X10^{-0})$	0.0	14.0	$1X10^{-14}$
	$1X10^{-1}$	1.0	13.0	$1X10^{-13}$
Gastric Juice	$1X10^{-2}$	2.0	12.0	$1X10^{-12}$
	$1X10^{-3}$	3.0	11.0	$1X10^{-11}$
Wine	$1X10^{-4}$	4.0	10.0	$1X10^{-10}$
Banana	$1X10^{-5}$	5.0	9.0	$1X10^{-9}$
	$1X10^{-6}$	6.0	8.0	$1X10^{-8}$
Milk	$1X10^{-7}$	7.0	7.0	$1X10^{-7}$
Seawater	$1X10^{-8}$	8.0	6.0	$1X10^{-6}$
Borax	$1X10^{-9}$	9.0	5.0	$1X10^{-5}$
	$1X10^{-10}$	10.0	4.0	$1X10^{-4}$
Lime water	$1X10^{-11}$	11.0	3.0	$1X10^{-3}$
	$1X10^{-12}$	12.0	2.0	$1X10^{-2}$
	$1X10^{-13}$	13.0	1.0	$1X10^{-1}$
Sodium Hydroxide (NaOH), 0.1M	$1X10^{-14}$	14.0	0.0	$1\ (1X10^{-0})$

Acidic ↑ / Basic ↓

Rubric 3: Basic Science Questions

1. What are the three distinct layers of tissue (from the surface to internal) that make up the skin?

    A) Dermis, Epidermis & Subcutaneous layer.
    B) Epidermis, Dermis & Subcutaneous layer.
    C) Subcutaneous layer, Epidermis & Dermis.
    D) Subcutaneous layer, Dermis & Epidermis.

2. Atopic people are predisposed to developing dermatitis. Why is this the case?

    A) Their reduced skin resistance to chemical irritants.
    B) Inherent dry skin and dysfunctional sweating.
    C) A high skin colonization rate of the bacterium Staphylococcus aureus.
    D) A & D.
    E) All of the above.

3. What are the three main categories to help determine what glove to select?

    A) Glove material used, type of work being done and type of hazard encountered.
    B) Glove material used, type of work being done and duration of glove use.
    C) Type of work being done, duration of glove use and type of hazard encountered.
    D) Type of work being done, type of hazard encountered and ambient temperature.

4. What determines the "fate" of an inhaled air contaminant?

    A) Size, Solubility & Concentration.
    B) Solubility, Concentration & Chemical reactivity.
    C) Size, Solubility & Chemical reactivity.
    D) Solubility, Concentration & pH.

5. What are the categories of inhaled contaminants that adversely affect the lungs?

    A) Dusts, Toxic Gases & Aerobes.
    B) Toxic aerosols, Toxic gases & Aerobes.
    C) Dust, Toxic gases & Toxic aerosols.
    D) Dust, Toxic aerosols & Aerobes.

6. Choose the answer that lists the layers of tissue surrounding the transparent internal structures of the eyeball.

    A) External fibrous layer and middle vascular layer.
    B) External fibrous layer and inner layer of nerve tissue.
    C) External fibrous layer, middle vascular layer and inner layer of nerve tissue.
    D) Inner layer of nerve tissue and middle vascular layer.

7. What important variables affect visual acuity?

   A) Luminance, position in the visual field, duration and contrast.
   B) Duration and contrast.
   C) Luminance, duration and contrast.
   D) Position in the visual field, duration and contrast.

8. Choose the answer that correctly lists the different types of radiation welding arcs create.

   A) Ultraviolet (UV) radiation, Visible light and Infrared (IR) radiation.
   B) Ultraviolet (UV) radiation, Ionizing radiation and Infrared (IR) radiation.
   C) Ultraviolet (UV) radiation, Visible light and Neutron radiation.
   D) Alfa particle radiation, Visible light and Infrared (IR) radiation.

9. Failure of the Eustachian tube to ventilate creates a vacuum in the middle ear space. This causes pathological events to occur. What is/are the pathological event(s)?

   A) Pulls fluid into the middle ear (Nonsuppurative otitis media).
   B) Pulls fluid out of the middle ear.
   C) Pulls the eardrum inward (retraction).
   D) Pulls the eardrum outward.
   E) A and B only.
   F) A and C only.
   G) All of the above.

10. Sensorineural hearing loss causes impairment to what anatomical components/part(s) of the ear?

   A) Cochlea.
   B) Oval window.
   C) Auditory nerve.
   D) A and B only.
   E) A and C only.
   F) B and C only.
   G) All of the above.

11. Using your knowledge on how to calculate molecular weight using the periodic table, find the molecular weight of ethanol (C_2H_6O).

   A) 46.068 g/mol.
   B) 29.018 g/mol.
   C) 193.682 g/mol.
   D) 44.984 g/mol.

12. A vapor is different from a gas in which of the following ways?

    A) Gases are materials that are in the gaseous state at normal temperature and pressure, whereas a vapor is a partially gaseous phase that exists in chemicals that are liquids at normal temperature and pressure.

    B) Vapors are materials that are in the gaseous state at normal temperatures and pressure, whereas a gas is a partially gaseous phase that exists in chemicals that are liquids at normal temperature and pressure.

    C) There is no difference between a gas and a vapor; they are interchangeable words that describe the same state of matter.

    D) A vapor is the term used to describe a denser gas.

13. Which of the following terms describes a liquid in which a solute can be dissolved?

    A) Vapor phase.
    B) Solvent.
    C) Solution.
    D) Acid.

14. Which of the following chemicals reacts dangerously with moisture in the air?

    A) Chlorine.
    B) Silane.
    C) Ammonia.
    D) Rhenium hexafluoride.

15. The appropriate personal protective clothing for handling sulfuric acid would be made of:

    A) Butyl rubber.
    B) Nitrile.
    C) Latex.
    D) A thick natural fiber such as wool or cotton.

16. The vapor pressure of any chemical compound is directly related to:

    A) Density.
    B) Solubility.
    C) Temperature.
    D) Boiling point.

17. An open 500 mL beaker of benzene (C_6H_6) evaporates in a research lab storage room. The room is unoccupied, the door is closed, and there is no ventilation. The room is 8 feet x 8 feet x 8 feet. Calculate the airborne room concentration assuming complete evaporation. The density of benzene is 0.876 g/mL.

    A) 9469 ppm.
    B) 10,200 ppm.
    C) 102 ppm.
    D) 947 ppm.

18. An IH trained in phase contrast microscopy is analyzing a filter for asbestos fiber density on the filter. Calculating the fiber density is the first of a two-step method for determining the airborne fiber concentration. If the fiber density is greater than 1300 f/mm^2, the results are reported as uncountable or probably biased. The sample for asbestos was collected over 450 minutes of an 8-hour shift at 2 L/m. After counting 100 fields, the average fiber count is 3 fibers per field. The field blank contains 0.01 fibers per field. It is known that the area of a 25 mm filter is 385 mm^2 and that the area of a graticule field is approximately 0.00785 mm^2. What is the fiber density, and is the sample acceptable?

    A) 1400 f/mm^2 and not acceptable.
    B) 381 f/mm^2 and acceptable.
    C) 3 f/mm^2 and not acceptable.
    D) 242 f/mm^2 and acceptable.

19. An IH trained in phase contrast microscopy is analyzing a filter for airborne asbestos fiber concentration. The sample for asbestos was collected over 450 minutes of an 8-hour shift at 2 L/m. After counting 100 fields, the average fiber count is 3 fibers per field. The field blank contains 0.01 fibers per field. It is known that the area of a 25 mm filter is 385 mm^2, and that the area of a graticule field is approximately 0.00785 mm^2. What is the fiber density, and is the sample acceptable?

    A) 147 f/mL or 147 f/cc.
    B) 0.33 f/mL or 0.33 f/cc.
    C) 1 f/mL or 1 f/cc.
    D) 0.16 f/mL or 0.16 f/cc.

20. Mercury vapor is best absorbed by which of the following?

    A) Treated amorphous silica.
    B) Activated charcoal impregnated with copper sulfate.
    C) Activated charcoal impregnated with iodine.
    D) Activated amorphous silica.

21. Which of the following is not functioning as a solvent in the application described?

    A) Xylene for paint clean-up.
    B) Ketones for spraying paint.
    C) Chlorinated hydrocarbons for cleaning parts.
    D) Epoxy for making foundry cores.

22. Calculate the amount of liquid in mL (SG 83, MW 100) that must be vaporized in a 5 x 5 x 4 feet chamber to create a concentration of 100 ppm:

    A) 1.4 mL.
    B) 1.9 mL.
    C) 14 mL.
    D) 19 mL.

23. The pressure in a closed vessel is doubled as a result of heating. The original temperature was 25°C. Calculate the new temperature.

    A) 50°C.
    B) 596°K.
    C) 461°R.
    D) 250°K.

24. What is the molar volume of a gas at 300°C and 0.95 atm?

    A) 49.5 L.
    B) 283 L.
    C) 44 L.
    D) 120 L.

25. A chemical has a molecular weight of 88. Where would the material likely accumulate?

    A) Floor.
    B) Ceiling.
    C) Mix uniformly.
    D) Unknown.

Rubric 3: Basic Sciences Answers

1. Answer B.
   Explanation: Three distinct layers of tissue make up the skin from the surface to internal: the epidermis, the dermis, and the subcutaneous layer. *Source: Fundamentals of Industrial Hygiene 5th Edition*

2. Answer E.
   Explanation: Atopic people are predisposed to developing dermatitis because of their reduced skin resistance to chemical irritants, inherent dry skin, dysfunctional sweating, and a high skin colonization rate of the bacterium Staphylococcus aureus. *Source: Fundamentals of Industrial Hygiene 5th Edition*

3. Answer A.
   Explanation: Categories of glove standards depend on the type of glove material used, type of work being done, and type of hazard encountered. *Source: Fundamentals of Industrial Hygiene 5th Edition*

4. Answer C.
   Explanation: The fate of an inhaled air contaminant depends on its size, solubility, and chemical reactivity. *Source: Fundamentals of Industrial Hygiene 5th Edition*

5. Answer C.
   Explanation: Inhaled contaminants that adversely affect the lungs fall into <u>three general categories:</u>
   -*Aerosols and dusts*, which, when deposited in the lungs, may produce tissue reaction and/or disease.
   -*Toxic gases* that may produce direct tissue injury.
   -*Toxic aerosols or gases* that do not affect the lung tissue, but are passed from the lung into
   the bloodstream, where they are carried to other organs or have adverse effects on the oxygen-carrying capacity of the bloodstream.
   Source: Fundamentals of Industrial Hygiene 5th Edition

6. Answer C.
   Explanation: The eyeball consists of three coats, or layers, of tissue surrounding the transparent internal structures. These layers consist of an external fibrous layer, a middle vascular layer, and an inner layer of nerve tissue. *Source: Fundamentals of Industrial Hygiene 5th Edition*

7. Answer A.
   Explanation: Important variables that affect visual acuity include luminance, position in the visual field, duration and contrast. *Source: Fundamentals of Industrial Hygiene 5th Edition*

8. Answer A.

    Explanation: Welding arcs give off radiation over a broad range of wavelengths - from 200 nm (nanometers) to 1,400 nm (or 0.2 to 1.4 µm, micrometers). This includes ultraviolet (UV) radiation (200 to 400 nm), visible light (400 to 700 nm), and infrared (IR) radiation (700 to 1,400 nm). UV-radiation is divided into three ranges - UV-A (315 to 400 nm), UV-B (280 to 315 nm) and UV-C (100 to 280 nm). UV-C and almost all UV-B are absorbed in the cornea of the eye. UV-A passes through cornea and is absorbed in the lens of the eye. Some UV radiation, visible light, and IR radiation can reach the retina.
    Source: https://www.ccohs.ca/oshanswers/safety_haz/welding/eyes.html

9. Answer F.

    Explanation: Failure of the Eustachian tube to ventilate creates a vacuum in the middle ear space, which in turn causes one of two pathological events to occur; it pulls fluid into the middle ear, resulting in a condition called nonsuppurative otitis media, or it pulls the eardrum inward (retraction). *Source: Fundamentals of Industrial Hygiene 5th edition*

10. Answer E.

    Explanation: Sensorineural hearing loss is the hearing difficulty caused by inner ear damage. "Sensori" refers to the sense organ in the inner ear, and "neural" refers to the nerve fibers. Sensorineural can involve impairment of the cochlea, the auditory nerve, or both. *Source: Fundamentals of Industrial Hygiene 5th edition*

11. Answer A.

    Explanation: The atomic weight of carbon is 12.011 g/mol, the atomic weight of hydrogen is 1.0079 g/mol, and the atomic weight of oxygen is 15.999 g/mol. To calculate the molecular weight, add together the atomic weight of each element, and make sure to use each element every time it appears in the molecular equation.

12. Answer A.

    Explanation: *Gas* – A state of matter in which the material has very low density and viscosity, can expand and contract greatly in response to changes in temperature and pressure, easily diffuses into other gases, and readily and uniformly distributes itself through any container. A gas can be changed to the liquid or solid state only by the combined effect of increased pressure and decreased temperature (below the critical temperature).
    Vapors – The gaseous form of substances that are normally in the solid or liquid state (at room temperature and pressure). The vapor can be changed back to the solid or liquid state by increasing the pressure or degreasing the temperature alone. Vapors also diffuse. Evaporation is the process by which a liquid is changed to the vapor state and mixed with the surrounding air. Solvents with low boiling points volatize readily. *Source: Fundamentals of Industrial Hygiene 5th edition*

13. Answer B.

    Explanation: Solvent - a substance that dissolves another substance. *Source: Fundamentals of Industrial Hygiene 5th edition*

14. Answer D.

   Explanation: Rhenium hexafluoride (e.g., liquid metal halide) reacts rapidly with moisture in the air. *Source: Fundamentals of Industrial Hygiene 5th edition*

15. Answer A.

   Explanation: According to Ansell Chemical Resistance Guide, butyl rubber glove material has an "excellent" degradation rating and a "good protection" permeation rating with a breakthrough time of 240-480 minutes. Nitrile glove material has a "not recommended" degradation rating and a "splash protection" permeation rating with a breakthrough time of 30-60 minutes. Latex and wool, or cotton, are not recommended for handling sulfuric acid.

16. Answer C.

   Explanation: Vapor pressure – Pressure (measured in pounds per square inch absolute-psia) exerted by vapor. If a vapor is kept in confinement over its liquid so that the vapor can accumulate above the liquid (the temperature being held constant), the vapor pressure approaches a fixed limit called the maximum (or saturated) vapor pressure, dependent only on the temperature and the liquid. *Source: Fundamentals of Industrial Hygiene 5th edition*

17. Answer A.

   Explanation:

   Step 1: Calculate the mass of the benzene spill

   $$500 \text{ mL} \times 0.876 \text{ g/mL} = 438 \text{ g or } 438000 \text{ mg}$$

   Step 2: Calculate the room volume

   $$8 \times 8 \times 8 = 512 \text{ ft}^3$$

   $$512 \text{ ft}^3 \times \frac{0.0283 m^3}{1 ft^3} = 14.5 \text{m}^3$$

   Step 3: Calculate the concentration in the room

   $$\frac{438000 \text{mg}}{14.5 m^3} = 30207 \frac{mg}{m^3}$$

   Convert to ppm assuming 25°C and 760 mmHg

   $$\text{ppm} = \frac{30207 mg/m^3 \ (24.45)}{78}$$
   $$= 9469 \text{ ppm}$$

18. Answer B.

   Explanation: Calculate and report fiber density on the filter, E (fibers/mm²), by dividing the average fiber count per graticule field, F/N$_f$, minus the mean field blank count per graticule field, B/N$_b$, by the graticule field area, A$_f$, (approx. 0.00785 mm²):

$$E_{fiber\ density} = \frac{\dfrac{F}{N_f} - \dfrac{B}{N_b}}{A_f}$$

Where:
E$_{fiber\ density}$ is amount of fibers on the filter in fibers/mm².
f/N$_f$ is the average or mean fiber count per graticule field.
B/N$_b$ is the mean fiber count per graticule field of the blank.
A$_f$ is the graticule field area (approximately 0.00785 mm^2).

$$E_{fiber\ density} = \frac{3 - 0.01\ fibers}{0.00785\ mm^2}$$
$$E_{fiber\ density} = 381\ f/mm^2$$

NOTE: Fiber counts above 1300 fibers/mm² and fiber counts from samples with >50% of filter area covered with particulate should be reported as "uncountable" or "probably biased." Other fiber counts outside the 100–1300 fiber/mm² range should be reported as having "greater than optimal variability" and as being "probably biased." *Source: NIOSH 7400*

19. Answer D.

   Explanation: The formula used to calculate the airborne concentration of fibers with the fiber density calculation in the numerator:

$$C_{asb} = \frac{(C_s - C_b)A_c}{1000\ (A_f)(V_s)}$$

Where:
C$_{asb}$ is the concentration of fibers in air (f/ml). f is airborne fibers. ml is mililiter.
C$_s$ is the average number of fibers counted per graticule field in the sample cassette filter.
C$_b$ is the average number of fibers counted per graticule field in the blank cassette filter.
V$_s$ is the volume of sampled air in liters.
A$_f$ is the approximate field area of the graticule – roughly 0.00785 mm$^{2.}$
A$_c$ is considered the effective collection area of the filter - roughly 385 mm^2 for a 25 mm diameter film.

$$V_s = 450\ minutes \times 2\ L/m = 900\ L$$

$$C_{asb} = \frac{(3 - 0.01\ fibers)385mm^2}{1000\frac{mL}{L}\ (0.00785mm^2)(900\ L)}$$

$$C_{asb} = 0.16\ f/mL\ and\ since\ mL\ and\ cc\ are\ equivalent\ 0.16\ f/cc$$

20. Answer C.
    Explanation: Mercury will volatilize from activated charcoal unless it is impregnated with Iodine. The mercury will bind with Iodine as Hg_2I_2 or HgI_2, which is more stable.

21. Answer D.
    Explanation: The epoxy reaction is polymerization and not solvent action.

22. Answer A.
    Explanation:
    Step 1: Calculate the volume of the chamber in Liters.
$$Volume = 5 \times 5 \times 4 \text{ feet}$$
$$Volume = 1000 \text{ ft}^3$$
$$1000 \text{ ft}^3 \times 28.3 \text{ L/ft}^3 = 2830 \text{ ft}^3$$

Step 2: Calculate the amount of liquid required for a target concentration of 100 ppm.

$$2830 \text{ L} \times \frac{100\ L\ chemical}{1,000,000\ L\ container} \times \frac{1\ g-mole\ chemical}{24.45\ L} \times \frac{100\ g}{1\ g-mole} \times \frac{1\ mL}{0.83\ g}$$
$$= 1.4 \text{ mL}$$

23. Answer B.
    Explanation: The volume remains constant.
    Step 1: Convert temperature to absolute

$$25 + 273 = 298°K$$

Step 2: Solve for T

$$\frac{P_1}{T_1} = \frac{P_2}{T_2}$$

$$\frac{1}{298} = \frac{2}{X}$$

$$X = 298 \times 2$$

$$X = 596$$

24. Answer A.

Explanation:

Step 1: Convert to absolute

$$300°C + 273°C = 573°C$$

Using the ideal gas law solve for V1

$$\frac{V_1 x (P_1)}{T_1} = \frac{P_2 x V_2}{T_2}$$

$$\frac{22.4 x (1)}{273} = \frac{.95 x V_2}{573}$$

$$V_2 = \frac{22.4\ x(573)}{273 x .95}$$

$$V_2 = 49.5\ L$$

25. Answer A.

Explanation: Molecular weight of air is approximately 30 gm/mole. Density of gas is directly proportional to molecular weight. Therefore, a gas of molecular weight of 88 gm/mole will sink.

Rubric 4: Biohazards

A biohazard is an agent capable of interacting with living cells or tissues and as a result of that interaction propagating itself or its effects.

Industries and professions where biological agents may present recognized hazards include health care; police and emergency services; clinical laboratories; agriculture and veterinary science; in-vitro diagnostic laboratories; medical device manufacturers; biotechnology; biological R&D; detergent enzymes and construction; or demolition of moldy infrastructure.

Biosafety programs are needed to enable the advancement of science and innovation in a safe and controlled manner.

To recognize, evaluate, and control biohazardous agents, one must recognize the different categories and nomenclature. There are seven different categories of biohazardous agents (see table below).

Table: Categories of Biohazard Agents

Agent Category	Defining Characteristics	Occupationally Important Examples
Bacteria	Bacteria are the oldest and most abundant life forms on Earth. They exist in three (3) main morphologies: spherical (cocci), rod-shaped (bacilli), spiral (spirilla). Bacteria are one cell microbes lacking chlorophyll and grow by simple division. Unlike the eukaryotes, bacterial cells are prokaryotes that lack a nucleus.	Escherichia coli pathogenic strains such as E. coli O157:H7, dubbed the "flesh eating" bacteria. Found in foods contaminated with fecal matter, destroys human cells and can cause fatal bleeding of the colon, bowel and kidneys. TB, or tuberculosis, a lung disease caused by Mycobacterium tuberculosis. TB is spread from human reservoir by droplet nuclei from coughing and sneezing.
Fungi	Fungi include mushrooms, molds and yeast, which are distinguishable from plants in that they do not make their own food. Occupationally important fungi get their nutrition by breaking down the remains of old dead plants or necrosing tissue in at-risk patients.	Aspergillus species are commonly found degrading organic matter in nature. A. fumigatus and A. flavus are opportunistic human pathogens, causing Aspergillosis in immunocompromised (AIDS, transplant) patients. Histoplasmosis, a systemic mycosis caused by Histoplasma capsulatum infection, typically as the result of the disturbance of bird or bat droppings.
Parasites	Single or multicellular organisms living on or in a host from which they derive sustenance without providing benefit. In biohazard parlance, parasites are assumed to be detrimental if not wholly pathogenic.	Toxoplasmosis caused by the coccidian protozoan of cats, Toxoplasma gondii. This agent may be spread via contaminated domestic cat feces to pregnant women, thus leading to fetal infection and death. Trichinellosis, caused by an intestinal roundworm, Trichinella spiralis. Spread by consumption of poorly cooked foods, especially pork.
Prions	Proteinaceous infectious particles that lack nucleic acids: composed largely of an abnormal isoform of a normal cellular protein.	Creutzfeldt-Jakob disease, a fatal degenerative brain disease. Bovine spongiform encephalopathy, or "mad cow disease", known to affect only cows at this time.
Rickettsia	Eubacteria, very small gram negative intracellular parasite is non-spore forming, and non-encapsulated. Lives in the cells of ticks and mites.	Clinically similar diseases transmitted by hard ticks, such as Rocky Mountain Spotted Fever caused by Rickettsia rickettsii and Queensland Tick Typhus caused by R. australis.
Viruses Other than Arboviruses	Ultramicroscopic pathogenic infectious agents characterized by multiplying in connection with living cells. Found in all living things, including bacteria and fungi. They are not presently considered cells, as they cannot carry out life functions independently.	Common colds, warts, Influenza, Viral Hepatitis A, B, C, D, and E. Herpesviruses, Poliovirus, and Rabies virus.
Arboviruses	Viruses transmitted by or borne by insects.	West Nile Fever, caused by the West Nile virus spread by mosquitoes preying on birds. Ebola virus, has caused 70% fatal outbreaks in equatorial Africa in 1995.

Recognition and Evaluation of Biological Hazards

Biological plausibility, the pathway of infection, and the association between the agent, host, and environment are important concepts. Biological plausibility is the concept that considers if the symptoms, complaints or conditions are consistent with known biological premises. Knowing the pathway of infection is critical in controlling the hazard. Breaking one or more links in a pathway of infection can prevent the spread of disease. If the biological hazardous agent actually enters the host in sufficient numbers constituting an infectious dose, and if the host is susceptible, infection can occur. A breakdown of biological hazard risk to humans and descriptions is represented in the table below.

Table: Biological Hazard Risk Levels to Humans

Level of Risk	*Description*
High Risk	Pose high risk of life-threatening disease, and there may be no known vaccine or treatment
Moderate Risk	Indigenous or exotic agents with potential for difficult-to-control airborne transmissions, and may produce diseases with serious or lethal consequences
Low Risk	Associated with human disease but unlikely to be fatal. Mostly spread via direct contact. There are usually curative medical treatments
Least Risk	Not known to cause disease in healthy adults

Control of Biological Hazards

Biological hazards are controlled through regulation of biological hazards, utilization of the biosafety levels, and engineering controls (e.g., biological safety cabinets). No standard regulation method exists when assessing risk of biological hazards to humans, but the specific agent involved is the first factor considered. Guidelines and standards of practice are safeguards for biological hazard exposure and control.

Approaches to biological safety are derived from biosafety programs. Regardless of the specific biosafety program, the main goal of every program is containment. Containment is broken down into primary and secondary barrier categories. Primary barriers describe controls to protect the worker and the immediate work area from potential exposure. Secondary barriers refer to the protection aimed at the external environment.

Biological safety cabinets (BSC) are effective engineering controls when working with biological hazards. BSC are designed to protect the cabinet user and those in the secondary environment from airborne biohazard exposures.

Education about and the utilization of biosafety levels (BSL) is crucial to effectively control biological hazards. This biohazard control model categorizes biohazards relative to the degree of hazard for specific operations. There are four biosafety levels that describe combinations of laboratory practices and techniques, equipment, and facility design features recommended for operations involving hazardous agents. The four biosafety levels are described in the table below.

Table: Biosafety Levels

Biosafety Level	*Description*
Level One	• Basic level of contaminant • Relies on standard microbiological work practices • For work with agents that are low risk and not known to cause disease in healthy adult humans
Level Two	• For work with moderate-risk agents that are normally present in the community • Can result in human disease • Primary hazards are accidental ingestion or contact exposures • Not known to be transmissible by the aerosol route • Protect against direct droplet exposures
Level Three	• Bio-agents that are aerosol transmissible, and either indigenous or exotic • Can cause serious or lethal human disease for which preventive or therapeutic interventions may be available • These agents pose high individual risk upon direct exposure, but low community risk upon release
Level Four	• Exotic biological agents that pose a high risk of life-threatening disease • Preventive or therapeutic interventions are not usually available • May be spread as an aerosol or possess an unknown risk of transmission

Decontamination, disinfection, and sterilization are alternative techniques for controlling biological hazards. Decontamination may be accomplished by physical means such as physically removing the hazard, or by chemical cleaning (soap, etc.).

Chemical disinfectants inactivate microorganisms by chemical reaction. The effectiveness of the disinfectant against an infectious agent varies with the nature of the chemical; the concentration; contact duration; temperature; humidity; pH; and the presence of organic material. Sterilization kills all forms of life, which is accomplished by heat, gases, irradiation or chemicals.

Table: Decontamination Techniques - Physical

Technique	Description
Steam	• Approximately 250°F under pressure (15-18 psi) • Most common and convenient method of sterilization
Wet Heat	• Boiling (212°F for > 30 minutes) • Pasteurization (161°F for 15 seconds, or 143°F for 30 minutes) kills vegetative cells but not bacterial spores • High temperature denatures enzymes and kills organisms
Dry Heat	• Open flames and Bacti-Cinerators ™ are used to sterilize inoculation loops • Ovens (air heated to 160-180°C for 2 hours) are used for anhydrous materials • Incinerators are used to destroy infectious waste material
Ionizing Radiation	• Used for the sterilization of new, prepackaged medical devices • Bulk package sterilization in the delivery of food
Ultraviolet (UV) Radiation	• Inactivate viruses, mycoplasma, bacteria and fungi • Also used in air locks, animal holding areas, and laboratory rooms, when not occupied • Least effective method of sterilization • Not practical for use with liquids
Filtration	• Membrane filters are used to remove bacteria, yeast and molds from solutions

Table: Decontamination Techniques - Chemical

Disinfectant Technique	Target Biological Hazard(s)
Iodophors (iodine-carrier)	• Antimicrobial and antiviral • Antiseptic and disinfectant purposes • Povidone-iodine is sporicidal and important in preventing wound infections
Glutaraldehyde	• Bacteria and their spores, mycelia and spore forms of fungi, and various viruses
Formaldehyde	• Vegetative bacteria, spores and viruses
Ozone	• Water purification
Sodium hypochlorite	• Bacteria, viruses and fungi
Alcohols	• Rapid acting bactericide, but do not destroy spores
Quaternary Ammonium Compounds	• General use disinfectants to control vegetative bacteria and nonlipid-containing viruses • Not active against bacterial spores
Phenolic Compounds (0.5%-2%)	• Killing of vegetative bacteria • Tuberculosis, fungi, and lipid-containing viruses
Ethylene oxide (EtO)	• Inactivates microorganisms, including endospores or bacteria viruses
Chlorine Dioxide	• Antimicrobial agent • Sodium Chlorite (stabilized ClO_2): destroys anthrax spores

Important Terms and Concepts

Bacteria- A small and relatively simple organism found in soil, water and the alimentary tract of animals and man. Some cause diseases in man.

Biohazardous waste- Byproducts containing blood, bodily fluids, or recognizable body parts that present a substantial or potential hazard to human health or the environment when managed improperly.

Bioterrorism- The use of biological agents, such as pathogenic organisms or agricultural pests, for terrorist purposes.

Biological safety cabinet- Containment equipment that prevents the release and transmission of biological agents.

Biological agents- Any of the viruses, microorganisms, and toxic substances derived from living organisms and used as offensive weapons to produce death or disease in humans, animals and growing plants.

Biosafety- The art and science of maintaining a broken chain of infection.

Biosafety level- The rating of biohazard potential described in four degrees of severity: (1) BSL1 agents are low risk and not known to cause disease in healthy adult humans; (2) BSL2 agents are associated with agents known to cause human disease that can be moderately serious, and for which preventative or therapeutic interventions are often available; (3) BSL3 agents are indigenous or exotic with potential for infection following aerosol transmission. Agents are associated with serious or lethal human disease for which preventative or therapeutic interventions may not be available; (4) BSL4 organisms are dangerous/exotic agents that pose a high risk of life-threatening disease, and for which preventative or therapeutic interventions are not usually available.

Biotechnology- Techniques that use living organisms or parts of organisms to produce a variety of products (from medicines to industrial enzymes) to improve plants or animals to develop microorganisms to remove toxics from bodies of water, or act as pesticides.

Bloodborne pathogen- Pathogenic organism(s) present in human blood, or other potentially infectious body fluids, that can cause disease in humans (e.g., HBV and HIV).

Colonization- The state in which infection and establishment of an organism within a host has occurred without resulting in subclinical or clinical disease. Detectable presence of microbes.

Communicable disease- An infectious disease due to a specific agent or its toxic products.

Contamination- The presence of a biohazardous agent on the body or inanimate objects, including water and food.

Decontamination- Removal of harmful substances, such as noxious chemicals, harmful bacteria or other organisms, or radioactive material from exposed individuals, rooms and furnishings in buildings or the exterior environment.

Disinfection- The killing of infectious agents (except bacterial spores) below the level necessary to cause infection. Sanitizers are used on inanimate surfaces; antiseptics are used on the skin.

Enzyme- An agent that catalyzes a biological reaction that is not itself consumed in the reaction.

Etiologic agent- A biohazardous material capable of causing infection and subsequent disease.

Genetic engineering- A process of inserting new genetic information into existing cells in order to modify an organism for the purpose of changing one of its characteristics.

Herd immunity- Immunity shared by all or most members of a group or community, which reduces invasive capacity of infectious disease.

Infection- (1) Invasion of the body by a pathogenic organism with or without disease manifestation. (2) Pathological condition resulting from invasion of a pathogen.

Infectivity- Qualitative term used to describe the apparent ease by which an infectious agent is spread to a host.

Microbe- A microorganism, especially a bacterium of a pathogenic nature.

Mold- A downy or furry growth on the surface of organic matter, caused by fungi, especially in the presence of dampness or decay.

Pasteurization- Heat treatment of fluids at specified temperatures for specified durations to kill human pathogens.

Pathogenicity- The act of producing disease. The ability of an infectious agent to produce infection and disease.

Pathway- The course a chemical or pollutant takes from the source to the organism exposed.

Personal protective equipment (PPE) - Equipment designed to protect individuals from biohazards.

Primary barriers- Protection of the worker and environment in the immediate area of potential exposure. Biosafety cabinets, sealed centrifuge rotors, glove boxes, high efficiency particulate aerosols (HEPA)-filtered animal enclosures, and PPE are important primary barriers.

Prion- Any of a group of tiny infectious agents composed mainly or entirely of protein; though lacking in demonstrable nucleic acid, prions are capable of self-replication and are thought to be the cause of various degenerative diseases of the nervous system of vertebrates.

Risk assessment- The process of determining, either quantitatively or qualitatively, the probability and magnitude of an undesired event, and estimating the cost to human society or the environment in terms of morbidity, mortality or economic impact.

Risk communication- The exchange of information about health or environmental risk among risk assessors and managers, the general public, news media, interest groups, etc.

Secondary barriers- Protection of the external environment, including non-laboratory work areas and the outside community.

Sterilization- Kills all forms of life. Accomplished by heat, gases, irradiation, or chemicals.

Sanitized- Process of decreasing the overall count of microbes present on inanimate objects through chemical means exclusively.

Virulence- The quality of being virulent, or very poisonous, noxious. Malignant. The relative infectiousness of a microorganism causing disease.

Zoonosis- Diseases transmissible from animals to man under normal host-environment conditions.

Zoonotic infection- Disease transmissible from animals to man.

Rubric 4: Biohazard Questions

1. Which bacteria produces a heat stable toxin that can survive being boiled for 25 minutes in addition to tolerating salty conditions?

    A) Clostridium botulinum.
    B) Clostridium perfringens.
    C) Staphylococcus aureus.
    D) Helicobacter pylori.

2. Which of the following is useful and practical for viable microbial contamination reduction in the air in animal holding areas, ventilated cabinets, and non-occupied laboratories?

    A) Germicidal UV radiation.
    B) HVAC.
    C) Disposable particulate respirators.
    D) Ionizing radiation.

3. Disinfection means:

    A) Killing or removing all organisms.
    B) Using specialized cleansing techniques that destroy or prevent growth of organisms capable of infection.
    C) Halting the growth of all microorganisms.
    D) Removing microorganisms from other living organisms.

4. Which of the following statements is incorrect regarding universal precautions?

    A) It applies to all male and female bodily fluids, including urine, sweat, and breastmilk.
    B) It is defined as an approach to infection control.
    C) It is correct to treat that all bodily fluids as though they are infectious.
    D) Employee uniforms do not necessarily serve as personal protective equipment or satisfy universal precautions.

5. Commonly associated with hoofed animals, this infection is associated with skin lesions and can be fatal if untreated.

    A) E. Coli.
    B) Rhinovirus.
    C) Glanders.
    D) Anthrax.

6. Botulinum toxin interferes with nerve impulses by disrupting the release of _______ from the axon terminal.

   A) Norepinephrine.
   B) Adrenalin.
   C) Amphetamine.
   D) Acetylcholine.

7. Which of these methods is considered the "standard" for sampling airborne microorganisms?

   A) Petri dish.
   B) Membrane filter.
   C) Breather test.
   D) Multistage cascade impactor.

8. The correct calibrated flow of an N6 (Andersen-type) single stage impactor for an accurate bioaerosol air sample should be:

   A) 16.4 lpm.
   B) 28.3 lpm.
   C) 17.6 lpm.
   D) 9.0 lpm.

9. Exposure to _________________ is associated with the occurrence of byssinosis.

   A) Asbestos.
   B) Cotton dust.
   C) Crystalline silica.
   D) Formaldehyde.

10. What are the four main categories of physical and chemical disinfection?

   A) Heat, liquid disinfectants, vapors and gasses, and radiation.
   B) Wet heat, dry heat, electrical current, and sunlight.
   C) Halogenated solvents, organic solvents, soaps, and carbamates.
   D) Alcohol, phenol, formaldehyde, and glutaraldehyde.

11. Which of the following is not a basic principle to be followed by a competent professional conducting a mold assessment?

    A) Excessive mold growth in a living or work space is undesirable and should be addressed.
    B) An exposure assessment should be performed immediately to ensure no one is overexposed.
    C) Conduct a thorough, informed visual inspection of all areas with excessive mold growth.
    D) Removal of visible mold growth is the preferred method of remediation.

12. The health effects of biohazards include which of the following?

    A) Infectious diseases, scoliosis, allergies.
    B) Infectious diseases, pneumoconiosis, acute toxic effects.
    C) Acute toxic effects, allergies, infectious diseases.
    D) Pneumoconiosis, dermatitis, alveolitis.

13. There are several fungi associated with occupational illness, such as Coccidioidomycosis, which can lead to San Joaquin Valley Fever, and ____, which is associated with bird droppings.

    A) Histoplasma capsulatum.
    B) Penicillium albocoremium.
    C) Alternaria alternata.
    D) Aspergillus acidus.

14. Giardia lamblia is an organism that lives in a host and causes adverse effects. Select the best description of this organism.

    A) Toxin.
    B) Parasite.
    C) Fungi.
    D) Arbovirus.

15. The laboratory manipulation of genetic material using enzymes to join this material to different genetic material outside of a living cell and capable of replicating in a living cell is an example of:

    A) Bio-mastication.
    B) Recombinant DNA.
    C) Prion management.
    D) Organic tetanospasmin.

16. An allergic inflammatory reaction in the pulmonary system caused by exposure to organic dusts containing fungi or thermophilic bacteria is an example of:

    A) Arboviritis.
    B) Lung cancer.
    C) Hypersensitvity pneumonitis.
    D) Pneumococcal alveolitis.

17. Which of the following is not considered a primary barrier?

    A) Safety cups for centrifuges, biosafety cabinets.
    B) Sharps disposal containers, self-sheathing needles.
    C) High efficiency filtration on enclosures, eye and face protection.
    D) Safety showers, disinfectants.

18. Choose the statement that best describes wet heat decontamination.

    A) Membrane filters are used to remove bacteria, yeast, and molds from biologic and pharmaceutical solutions.
    B) Boil (212°F for > 30 minutes) and pasteurization (161°F for 15 seconds, or 143°F for 30 minutes) kills vegetative cells but not bacterial spores. High temperature causes denaturation of enzymes and kill organisms.
    C) Heat at 250°F under pressure (15-18 psi) in an autoclave. Most widely used and convenient method of sterilization.
    D) Inactivation of viruses, mycoplasma, bacteria, and fungi. Least effective and least perfected method of sterilization. Not practical as a disinfectant of liquids.

19. Choose the statement that best describes ionizing radiation decontamination.

    A) Boiling (212°F for > 30 minutes) and pasteurization (161°F for 15 seconds, or 143°F for 30 minutes) kills vegetative cells but not bacterial spores. High temperature cause denaturation of enzymes and kill organisms.
    B) Open flames and Bacti-Cinerators (tm) (an electrical device that dry-heats at 1600°F) are used to heat sterilize inoculation loops. Hot air ovens (160-180°C for 2 hours) are used for anhydrous materials (e.g., greases and powders). Incinerators are used to destroy infectious waste.
    C) Inactivation of viruses, mycoplasma, bacteria, and fungi. Least effective and least perfected method of sterilization. Not practical as a disinfectant of liquids.
    D) Sterilization of new, prepackaged medical devices (e.g., syringes and catheters) and in bulk package sterilization in the delivery of food industries.

20. Choose the statement that best describes filtration decontamination.

    A) Heat at 250°F under pressure (15-18 psi) in an autoclave. Most widely used and convenient method of sterilization.

    B) Membrane filters are used to remove bacteria, yeast, and molds from biologic and pharmaceutical solutions.

    C) Boil (212°F for > 30 minutes) and pasteurization (161°F for 15 seconds, or 143°F for 30 minutes) kills vegetative cells but not bacterial spores. High temperature cause denaturation of enzymes and kill organisms

    D) Sterilization of new, prepackaged medical devices (e.g., syringes and catheters) and in bulk package sterilization in the delivery of food industries.

Rubric 4: Biohazard Answers

1. Answer C.
   Explanation: Staphylococcus aureus produces a heat stable toxin that allows it to survive boiling for 25 minutes. It is also tolerant of salty environments.

2. Answer A.
   Explanation: Germicidal UV radiation is considered useful for small areas. *Source: Biohazards Reference Manual, AIHA*

3. Answer B.
   Explanation: Disinfection describes a process that eliminates many or all pathogenic microorganisms, except bacterial spores, on inanimate objects. *Source: CDC Guideline for Disinfection and Sterilization in Healthcare Facilities*

4. Answer A.
   Explanation: Universal precautions apply to blood, fluids in which blood is indistinguishably mixed, and bodily fluids which visibly contain blood; however, the examples in answer "A" are excluded from universal precautions unless they visibly contain blood.

5. Answer D.
   Explanation: While not usually fatal if treated, anthrax can cause skin lesions as well as respiratory problems for those who contract the infection. Workers in stock yards and those who work around hoofed animals are at risk of contracting the infection from infected animals.

6. Answer D.
   Explanation: Botulism derives from ingestion of uncooked anaerobic food, where spores of Clostridium botulinum have germinated with the production of the toxin (e.g., foodborne botulism). Botulinum toxin interferes with nerve impulses by disrupting the release of acetylcholine from the axon terminal. *Source: Montecucco, Cesare: The Mechanism of Action of Tetanus and Botulinum Neurotoxins*

7. Answer D.
   Explanation: The collection of airborne microorganisms is done by drawing air through a 400-hole sixth stage of a multistage cascade impactor. Air from each hole hits the medium, and bacterial or fungal can impact and eventually grow. *Source: Fundamentals of Industrial Hygiene, 5th Edition*

8. Answer B.
   Explanation: The correct calibrated flow of an N6 (Anderson-type) single stage impactor for an accurate bioaerosol air sample is 28.3 lpm. Source: N6 Single-Stage Viable Andersen Cascade Impactor User Manual

9. Answer B.

    Explanation: Brown lung disease – or byssinosis – is caused by long term exposure to cotton dust. Asbestos exposure can cause asbestosis and can lead to mesothelioma. Exposure to crystalline silica can cause silicosis.

10. Answer A.

    Explanation: Heat, liquid disinfectants, vapors and gasses, and radiation are the four main categories. Wet and dry heat are forms of heat utilized. Halogens, organic solvents and soaps are types of disinfectants. Carbamates are a type of pesticide. *Source: AIHA Biohazards Reference Manual*

11. Answer B.

    Explanation: According to the AIHA publication *Assessment, Remediation, and Post Remediation of MOLD in BUILDINGS*; answers A, C, and D are basic principles to be followed by a Competent Professional conducting a mold assessment.

12. Answer C.

    Explanation: The effects include acute toxic effects, allergies, and infectious diseases.

13. Answer A.

    Explanation: H. capsulatum is the agent responsible for histoplasmosis, a fungal disease of the lungs. Workers are exposed in cleaning operations and hatcheries. *Source: Intermountain Healthcare Biohazard Lecture*

14. Answer B.

    Explanation: G. lamblia is a protozoan parasite that causes intestinal disorders. *Source: Intermountain Healthcare Biohazard Lecture*

15. Answer B.

    Explanation: The question describes the recombinant DNA process. *Source: Intermountain Healthcare Biohazard Lecture*

16. Answer C.

    Explanation: Hypersensitivity is a set of undesirable reactions produced by the normal immune system, including allergies and autoimmunity. These reactions may be damaging, uncomfortable, or occasionally fatal. Pneumonitis is inflammation of the lungs.

17. Answer D.

    Explanation: Safety cups for centrifuges; biosafety cabinets; sharps disposal containers; self-sheathing needles; high efficiency filtration on enclosures; and eye and face protection are all examples of a primary barrier. Showers and disinfectants are administrative actions. *Source: Intermountain Healthcare Biohazard Lecture*

18. Answer B.
    Explanation: <u>Per the Physical Agent Decontamination table in this section.</u>
    Wet Heat: Boil (212°F for > 30 minutes) and pasteurization (161°F for 15 seconds, or
    143°F for 30 minutes) kills vegetative cells but not bacterial spores. High temperatures
    cause denaturation of enzymes and kill organisms. *Source: The Occupational Environment:
    Its Evaluation, Control, and Management, 3rd edition*

19. Answer: D
    Explanation: <u>Per the Physical Agent Decontamination table in this section.</u>
    Ionizing Radiation: Used for the sterilization of new, prepackaged medical devices and
    bulk package sterilization in the delivery of food. *Source: The Occupational Environment:
    Its Evaluation, Control, and Management, 3rd edition*

20. Answer: B
    Explanation: <u>Per the Physical Agent Decontamination table in this section.</u>
    Filtration: Membrane filters are used to remove bacteria, yeast, and molds from solutions.
    Source: The Occupational Environment: Its Evaluation, Control, and Management, 3rd edition

Rubric 5: Biostatistics and Epidemiology

Epidemiology

Epidemiology is the study of how a disease in a population is distributed and how particular factors influence this distribution. The main goal of epidemiology is to determine the causation of a particular disease. If the cause is unknown, epidemiologists strive to deliver insight on how a disease or injury arose and provide an explanation on how the disease or injury can be mitigated or eliminated. This is possible by studying a population at risk and determining what factors may lead to a particular disease.

Epidemiology is focused on a population perspective or groups of people, not individuals. The premise underlying epidemiology is that disease and illness are not randomly distributed in a population. Rather, each of us has certain characteristics that predispose us to, or protect us against, a variety of different diseases.

Epidemiology attempts to evaluate and analyze relationships that can reveal the cause of a disease. Determining a target population with the disease and understanding what risk factors or determinants are involved makes it possible to approximate the causation of the disease. Understanding these risk factors or determinants makes it easier to understand how a disease develops and how these risk factors or determinants can speed up or slow down the development of a particular disease.

Source: The Occupational Environment: Its Evaluation, Control and Management
Source: Epidemiology 5ᵗʰ Edition, Leon Gordis

Important Terms and Concepts

Case series- A descriptive study of common factors shared by a series of people with the same or similar outcome.

Epidemiology- The study of the distribution and determinants of disease frequency in a population.

Incidence- The number of individuals with an outcome in a population over a specified period of time that were outcome-free at the beginning of the time period (i.e. new cases).

Incidence rate- Number of new cases of disease per worker population per time period.

Occupational epidemiology- The study of the working population and the risks for illness and injury associated with the work environment.

Odds- The number of individuals with the outcome divided by the number without the outcome in the same exposure group.

Odds ratio- Approximation to relative risk for diseases of low frequency. (Number of cases with exposure times number of controls with no exposure) divided by (number of cases with no exposure times number of controls with exposure).

Person-time- The amount of time a person is at risk of developing an outcome, usually beginning at the time of first exposure to the suspected agent of risk.

Prevalence- The number of individuals with an outcome in a population over a specified period of time, including existing and new cases.

Prevalence rate- Number of existing cases of a disease in a worker population at a specified time.

Risk- The chance that an event will occur or a person in a group will get the outcome of interest.

- *Absolute risk-* The number of cases or people with an outcome in a population over a period of time.

- *Relative risk-* Prevalence rate of a disease in the exposed worker population divided by the prevalence rate of disease in the unexposed worker population.

- *Attributable risk-* Prevalence of disease in the exposed worker population minus the prevalence rate in the unexposed.

Statistics

The study of statistics encompasses the collection, organization, analysis, and interpretation of numerical data. When the focus is on biological and health sciences, the term biostatistics is commonly used. A working knowledge of statistics is crucial in evaluating the assumptions that statistical tools are based upon. These tools can support decision making and reduces the likelihood of interpreting the data incorrectly.

A statistic is a characteristic of a sample used to characterize the underlying population. A sample is the portion, part, or subset of the population used for observations and study. Sample data often are used to make inferences about the true values of population parameters. A parameter is a quantity that describes a statistical population. Common parameters include the sample mean and sample standard deviation.

Important Terms and Concepts

Alternative hypothesis- A condition different from the condition specified by the null hypothesis. For example, for audit, baseline, and surveillance surveys, the alternative hypothesis is that the exposure profile is unacceptable. For termination-reduction and commissioning surveys, the alternative hypothesis is that the exposure profile is acceptable.

Arithmetic mean- A measure of central tendency, calculated as the sum of all values in a population divided by the number of values in the population.

Central Limit Theorem- The sampling distribution of the mean approaches a normal distribution as the sample size increases, regardless of the shape of the underlying population distribution.

Coefficient of Variation- The sample standard deviation divided by the sample mean (or population parameters). When comparing variations between distributions with different means, coefficients of variation should be used. Sometimes expressed as a percentage. Abbreviated CV.

Confidence interval- A range of values (i.e., interval) that has a specified probability of including the true value of the parameter(s) of an underlying distribution.

Confidence limits- The upper and lower boundaries of a confidence interval. Upper confidence limit is abbreviated UCL; lower confidence limit is abbreviated LCL.

Decision statistic- An estimate of the parameter selected to represent the acceptability of an exposure profile. For example, the 95th percentile is often used as the decision statistic when comparing an exposure profile to an OEL.

Descriptive statistics- Simple metrics of a sample distribution's characteristics, such as central tendency (e.g., mean, median) and dispersion (e.g., standard deviation, variance, range). Other examples include number of samples and actual fraction of samples above an OEL. Contrast with inferential statistics.

Geometric mean- The nth root of the product of n values. The geometric mean is the median of lognormally distributed data. The geometric mean and arithmetic mean of most distributions are not equal and should not be used interchangeably. Arithmetic mean is the correct parameter for evaluating cumulative exposure.

Geometric standard deviation- The antilog of the standard deviation of the log transformed data (measure of variability for a lognormal distribution). A GSD of greater than 2 indicates large variability. A GSD of 1.44 or less indicates a that a data set may be approximated by the NORMAL distribution per NIOSH 1977.

Homogeneous- In statistics, having identical probability distribution functions.

Hypothesis test- A statistical test, based on a random sample from a population, which assigns a confidence level on a parameter of the population. In industrial hygiene, a hypothesis test will often be performed to compare summary measures of exposure data with standards or OELs.

Inferential statistics- Parameters used to make estimates about the exposure distribution and underlying population.

Lognormal distribution- The distribution of a random variable with the property such that the logarithms of its values are normally distributed.

Mean- The arithmetic average of a set of data and not used as a substitute for geometric mean.

Mean test- A statistical test that evaluates whether the sample arithmetic mean exposure equals a specified population mean value.

Measurement error- The difference between the true value and the value obtained by a measuring device. In the absence of systematic bias, the distribution of measurement errors is often considered measurement precision.

Median- The exposure measurement that divides a set of measurements into two equal parts, with half less than and half greater than this value.

Mode- The value in a set of measurements that occurs most frequently; the maximum value of a continuous probability density function. The mode of a lognormal distribution is less than the median, which is less than the mean. The mean, median, and mode of a normal distribution are equal.

Non-parametric- Statistical methods that do not assume a particular statistical distribution for the statistic of interest (e.g., distribution-free methods).

Normal distribution- An important symmetric probability distribution characterized completely by two parameters: the mean and the standard deviation. It has its highest ordinate at the center and tails off to zero in both directions, thus forming a bell-shaped curve.

Null hypothesis- The assumed or default condition. For example, for audit, baseline, and surveillance surveys, it is assumed that the exposure profile is acceptable. For termination-reduction and commissioning surveys, it is assumed that the exposure profile is unacceptable. The null hypothesis is considered correct unless there is compelling evidence that it is likely to be incorrect.

Parameter- A quantity that describes a statistical population (e.g., mean and standard deviation, geometric mean, geometric standard deviation).

Parametric- Statistical tests are said to be parametric if an underlying statistical distribution, described by appropriate parameters, is based solely on computations involving these parameters.

Population statistics- The true parameters calculated by including the entire population (e.g., population mean and standard deviation). In workplace exposure assessment, these parameters usually must be estimated from a representative sample of the population and, therefore, are not known exactly.

Probability paper- Graph paper on which a specific family of distributions is represented by spacing along a probability axis. For example, samples from a lognormal distribution appear as a straight line when plotted on log probability paper, and samples from a normal distribution appear as a straight line when plotted on linear-probability paper.

Range- The difference between the largest and smallest values in a measurement data set.

Sample- The portion, part, or subset of the population drawn for observation or the measurement chosen for statistical analysis and study. Sample data is often used to make inferences about the true values of population parameters.

Sample parameters- Estimators of population parameters based on observation of a subgroup of the population (e.g., sample means and sample standard deviation).

Standard deviation- The positive square root of the variance of a distribution; the parameter measuring spread of values about the mean. It can be estimated from the slope of the straight line through data plotted on probability paper.

Statistic- A characteristic of a sample, such as sample mean and sample standard deviation: used to characterize the underlying population.

Statistical power- One minus the probability that a given test causes acceptance of the null hypothesis; this is the same as the probability of rejecting the null hypothesis by a test when the alternative is true.

Statistical significance- The statistically based probability that the null hypothesis is true. If that probability is small (e.g., less than 5%) the null hypothesis is rejected.

Students t-distribution- A family of probability distributions distinguished by their degrees of freedom and used as the sampling distribution of arithmetic means when the population standard deviation is unknown. As sample size increases, the t-distribution approaches a normal distribution.

Variance- The mean of the square of the differences between the mean value of population and randomly selected values from the same population. Units are squares of the data units, such as cm^2 or m^2.

Examples

Mean

The mean is a measure of central tendency. It is the most commonly investigated characteristic of a set of data. The mean is calculated by summing all the observations in a set of data and dividing by the total number of measurements.

A group of employees at Company XYZ was studied to evaluate exposure to Methylene Chloride. The table shown lists the Acetone exposure levels for each employee. If X is used to represent MC_1, $X_1 = 2.5$ denotes the first in the series of observations; $X_2 = 3.8$, the second; and so on up through x_{15}.

$$\bar{X} = \frac{X_1 + X_2 + \cdots + X_n}{n}$$

Given:

$\bar{X}$ is the arithmetic mean for a set of data (observations or data points) obtained for a complete population or a sample of the population. The units are the same as the units of the data set.

$X_1, X_2, \ldots X_n$ are the individual values for each observation in the data set.

n is the total number of observations in the data set.

<u>Calculate the average or mean methylene chloride exposure levels.</u>

Table: Methylene Chloride Exposure

Employee	Methylene Chloride Exposure (ppm)
1	2.5
2	3.8
3	7.0
4	8.5
5	2.1
6	4.6
7	12.3
8	8.4

Answer: 6.15 ppm

Explanation:

$$\bar{X} = \frac{X_1 + X_2 + \cdots + X_n}{n}$$

$$\bar{\bar{X}} = \frac{2.5 + 3.8 + 7.0 + 8.5 + 2.1 + 4.6 + 12.3 + 8.4}{8}$$

$$\bar{X} = \frac{49.2}{8}$$

$$\bar{X} = 6.15 \; ppm$$

If you are using the TI 30X IIS, use the following calculation keystrokes:

Step 1

Set to STAT Mode using the second function of DATA key

Step 2

Select 1-VAR and Enter key

Step 3

Press DATA Key

Step 4

Enter Data (X_1, down arrow key, FRQ, down arrow key; X_2, down arrow key, FRQ, down arrow key; … X_n, down arrow key, FRQ, down arrow key)

Step 5

Press STATVAR key

Step 6

Use arrow keys and select $\bar{x}$

Source: Principles of Biostatistics 2nd Edition
Source: Industrial-Occupational Hygiene Calculations: A Professional Reference

Variance

The variance is commonly used to measure dispersion within a set of data. The variance quantifies the amount of variability around the mean. The variance is calculated by subtracting the mean of a set of values from each of the observations, squaring the deviations, adding the deviations up, and dividing by 1 less than the number of observations in the data set.

A group of employees were studied to evaluate their methylene chloride exposures. The table represents eight methylene chloride exposure levels. The mean is 6.15 ppm.

$$s^2 = \frac{1}{n} \sum_{i=1}^{n} (\bar{x} - x_i)^2$$

Given:

s^2 = the amount of variability, or spread, around the mean of the measurements
$\bar{x}$ = the mean of the set of values in the sample
x_i = the value of each "ith" member of the set of observations
n = the number of observations in the data set

Calculate the variance.

Table: Methylene Chloride Exposure

Employee	Methylene Chloride Exposure (x_i)	$(\bar{x} - x_i)$	$(\bar{x} - x_i)^2$
1	2.5	3.65	13.32
2	3.8	2.35	5.52
3	7.0	-0.85	0.72
4	8.5	-2.35	5.52
5	2.1	4.05	16.40
6	4.6	1.55	2.40
7	12.3	-6.15	37.82
8	8.4	-2.25	5.06
Total	49.2	0	86.76

Answer: 12.395 ppm^2

Explanation:
Step 1: Calculate the variance

$$s^2 = \frac{1}{(n-1)} \sum_{i=1}^{n} (\bar{x} - x_i)^2$$

$$s^2 = \frac{1}{(8-1)} \sum_{i=1}^{8} (6.15 - x_i)^2$$

$$s^2 = \frac{86.76}{7}$$

$$s^2 = 12.39 \; ppm^2$$

If you are using the TI 30X IIS, use the following calculation keystrokes:

Step 1

Set to STAT Mode using the second function of DATA key

Step 2

Select 1-VAR and Enter key

Step 3

Press DATA key

Step 4
Enter Data (X_1, down arrow key, FRQ, down arrow key; X_2, down arrow key, FRQ, down arrow key; … X_n, down arrow key, FRQ, down arrow key)

Step 5

Press STATVAR key

Step 6

Use arrow keys and select Sx

Step 7
Square the value
Source: Principles of Biostatistics 2nd Edition

Standard Deviation

The standard deviation of a set of data is the positive square root of the variance. The standard deviation is used more frequently than the variance because the standard deviation has the same units of measurement as the mean, rather than squared units. When comparing two groups of data, the group with the smaller standard deviation has the more consistent observations; the group with the larger standard deviation presents a greater amount of variability.

A study was conducted among a group of employees to evaluate their methylene chloride exposures. The table represents eight Methylene Chloride exposure levels. The mean is 6.15 *ppm*.

$$SD = \sqrt{\frac{\Sigma(\bar{x} - x_i)^2}{n - 1}}$$

Given:

SD is the sample standard deviation. It is a measure of the dispersion around the mean of the values in a sample or population. It has the same units as the values in the sample.
$\bar{x}$ is the mean of the set of values in the sample.
x_i is the value of each data point in the sample.
n is the total number of data points or observations.

Calculate the Standard Deviation.

Table: Methylene Chloride Exposure

Employee	Methylene Chloride Exposure (x_i)	$(\bar{x} - x_i)$	$(\bar{x} - x_i)^2$
1	2.5	3.65	13.32
2	3.8	2.35	5.52
3	7.0	-0.85	0.72
4	8.5	-2.35	5.52
5	2.1	4.05	16.40
6	4.6	1.55	2.40
7	12.3	-6.15	37.82
8	8.4	-2.25	5.06
Total	49.2	0	86.76

Answer: 3.52 ppm

Explanation:
Step 1: Calculate the standard deviation

$$SD = \sqrt{\frac{\Sigma(\bar{x} - x_i)^2}{n - 1}}$$

$$SD = \sqrt{\frac{\Sigma(6.15 - x_i)^2}{8 - 1}}$$

$$SD = \sqrt{\frac{86.76}{7}}$$

$$SD = 3.52 \; ppm$$

If you are using the TI 30X IIS, use the following calculation keystrokes:

Step 1

Set to STAT Mode using the second function of DATA key

Step 2

Select 1-VAR and Enter key

Step 3

Press DATA key

Step 4

Enter Data (X_1, down arrow key, FRQ, down arrow key; X_2, down arrow key, FRQ, down arrow key; … X_n, down arrow key, FRQ, down arrow key)

Step 5

Press the STATVAR key

Step 6

Use arrow keys and select Sx

Source: Principles of Biostatistics 2nd Edition
Source: Industrial-Occupational Hygiene Calculations: A Professional Reference

Coefficient of Variation

The coefficient of variation is a measure of the relative variation of a set of values from normally distributed data. The coefficient of variation enables comparison of the variability among two or more sets. The coefficient of variation relates the standard deviation to the mean and is the ratio of the standard deviation to the mean, multiplied by 100.

Example: A study was conducted among a group of employees to evaluate their methylene chloride exposures. The table represents eight Methylene Chloride exposure levels. The mean is 6.15 *ppm*.

$$CV = \frac{SD}{\bar{x}}$$

Given:

SD is the sample standard deviation, which is a measure of the dispersion of the values in a data set. It has the same units as the values in the sample.

$\bar{x}$ is the arithmetic mean of a data set. It has the same units as the observations that comprise the population or the sample.

CV is the measure of the relative variation. It is expressed as a percentage or a decimal fraction of 1.

Calculate the coefficient of variation.

Table: Methylene Chloride Exposure

Employee	Methylene Chloride Exposure (ppm)
1	2.5
2	3.8
3	7.0
4	8.5
5	2.1
6	4.6
7	12.3
8	8.4
Total	49.2

Answer: 57%

Explanation:

Table: Coefficient of Variation

Employee	Methylene Chloride Exposure (x_i)	$(\bar{x} - x_i)$	$(\bar{x} - x_i)^2$
1	2.5	3.65	13.32
2	3.8	2.35	5.52
3	7.0	-0.85	0.72
4	8.5	-2.35	5.52
5	2.1	4.05	16.40
6	4.6	1.55	2.40
7	12.3	-6.15	37.82
8	8.4	-2.25	5.06
Total	49.2	0	86.76

Step 1: Calculate the Coefficient of Variation

$$CV = \frac{SD}{\bar{x}}$$

$$CV = \frac{3.52\ ppm}{6.15\ ppm}$$

$$CV = 0.57 \times 100$$

$$CV = 57\%$$

Source: Principles of Biostatistics 2nd Edition
Source: Industrial-Occupational Hygiene Calculations: A Professional Reference

Geometric Mean (log form)

The geometric mean is a measure of the central tendency of a distribution of values. The geometric mean can be calculated by taking the antilog of the log-transformed values divided by the number of values (n).

$$GM = 10^{\frac{\Sigma(log x)}{n}}$$

Terms and Units:

GM is the geometric mean of a data set. It has the same units as the values that comprise the population.

log x is the base 10 logarithm of the value of each data point.

n is the number of data points in the data set.

A set of 15 air samples was collected for measurement of exposure to toluene. The results are 11 ppm, 14 ppm, 19 ppm, 22 ppm, 26 ppm, 29 ppm, 32 ppm, 35 ppm, 38 ppm, 45 ppm, 56 ppm, 57 ppm, 61 ppm, 63 ppm, and 78 ppm.

Table: Geometric Mean (log form)

X_i (ppm)	Log X_i
11	1.04
14	1.14
19	1.28
22	1.34
26	1.41
29	1.46
32	1.51
35	1.54
38	1.58
45	1.65
56	1.75
57	1.76
61	1.79
63	1.80
78	1.90
$\Sigma \log x_i = 22.95$	

Calculate the geometric mean (log form).

Explanation:

Step 1: Calculate the sum of the base 10 logarithm of the values

Step 2: Calculate the geometric mean (log form)

$$GM = 10^{\frac{\Sigma(logx)}{n}}$$

$$GM = 10^{22.95/15}$$

$$GM = 33.88 \; ppm$$

Source: Industrial-Occupational Hygiene Calculations: A Professional Reference

Geometric Mean (nth root form)

The geometric mean (nth root form) is a measure of the central tendency of a distribution of values. The nth root method involves taking nth root of the product of the values in the data set from. The geometric mean is utilized when the range of values in the sample or population is large.

$$GM = \sqrt[n]{(x_1)(x_2)\dots(x_n)}$$

Terms and Units:

n is the number of data points in the data set.

GM is the geometric mean. It has the same units as the values that compromise the population.

$X_1, X_2, \dots X_n$ is the value of each data point in the data set.

A set of 15 air samples was collected for measurement of exposure to toluene. The results are 11 ppm, 14 ppm, 19 ppm, 22 ppm, 26 ppm, 29 ppm, 32 ppm, 35 ppm, 38 ppm, 45 ppm, 56 ppm, 57 ppm, 61 ppm, 63 ppm, and 78 ppm.

Table: Toluene Exposure

X_i (ppm)
11
14
19
22
26
29
32
35
38
45
56
57
61
63
78

Calculate the geometric mean (n^{th} root form).

Explanation:
Step 1: Calculate the geometric mean (n^{th} root form)

$$GM = \sqrt[n]{(x_1)(x_2)\dots(x_n)}$$

$$GM = \sqrt[15]{(11 \times 14 \times 19 \times 22 \times 26 \times 29 \times 32 \times 35 \times 38 \times 45 \times 56 \times 57 \times 61 \times 63 \times 78)}$$

GM = 33.88 *ppm*

Source: Industrial-Occupational Hygiene Calculations: A Professional Reference

Geometric Standard Deviation (84.13% Method)
A log-probability plot is one method to check the fit of a set of data to log normality. Also, a GSD of 1.44 or less indicates a that a data set may be approximated by the NORMAL distribution per NIOSH 1977. According to Gilbert (1987) if the ratio from the highest to lowest data point exceeds 20, then the data is likely skewed.

After creating the probability plot, the 50% probability of occurrence value corresponds to the median of the distribution, and the ratio of the 84.13% value to the 50% value corresponds to the geometric standard deviation (GSD).

$$GSD = \frac{84.13\ \%tile\ value}{50\ \%tile\ value}$$

Geometric Standard Deviation (15.87% Method)
After creating the probability plot, the 50% probability of occurrence value corresponds to the median of the distribution, and the ratio of the 50% value to the 15.87% value approximates the GSD.

$$GSD = \frac{50\ \%tile\ value}{15.87\ \%tile\ value}$$

Source: Industrial-Occupational Hygiene Calculations: A Professional Reference

Sampling and Analytical Error (SAE)

The measured exposure is unlikely to be the actual exposure due sampling and analytical errors (SAE). The uncertainty was addressed in the OSHA technical manual with the use of the one-sided (upper and lower) confidence limits. The sampling and analytical error (SAE) can be derived from the total coefficient of variation times the statistical constant (1.645), which is the statistical standard normal deviate for a one-sided 95% confidence limit. Refer to the z-table. The SAE is either a percentage or a decimal less than 1.

$$SAE = 1.645 \, CV_{total}$$

Example:

A sampling and analytical method for octane is reported to have a total coefficient of variation (CV_{total}) of 0.08 (or 8%).

Explanation:

The SAE for the method is

$$SAE = 1.654 \, CV_{total}$$

$$SAE = (1.645)(0.08)$$

$$SAE = 0.132$$

$$SAE = 0.132 \times 100 = 13.2\%$$

Source: Industrial-Occupational Hygiene Calculations: A Professional Reference

Pooled Standard Deviation

The pooled standard deviation combines information from both samples, which provides a more reliable estimate of the standard deviation. This gives the larger group a greater effect on the estimate.

$$SD_{pooled} = \sqrt{\frac{(n_1 - 1)SD_1{}^2 + (n_2 - 1)SD_2{}^2}{n_1 + n_2 - 2}}$$

Two groups of workers are selected from similar work areas in a lead acid battery manufacturing facility to compare the mean blood lead levels between the groups. The distribution is assumed normal and the variance assumed equal. The following results are obtained:

Method 1: mean = 18.9 ug/dL, SD = 5.9 ug/dL, n = 9
Method 2: mean = 11.9 ug/dL, SD = 6.3 ug/dL, n = 13

The pooled standard deviation may be used to perform a hypothesis test using the t-test. Based on the above, calculate the pooled standard deviation.

Step 1: Calculate the SD_{pooled}

$$SD_{pooled} = \sqrt{\frac{(n_1 - 1)SD_1{}^2 + (n_2 - 1)SD_2{}^2}{n_1 + n_2 - 2}}$$

$$SD_{pooled} = \sqrt{\frac{[(8)(5.9)^2 + (12)(6.3)^2]}{20}}$$

$$SD_{pooled} = 6.1 \text{ ug/dL}$$

Source: Principles of Biostatistics, Pagano, et al, 2nd edition

t-test & Hypothesis Testing
The t-test can be used to determine if the means from two sets of data are different from each other in a statistically significant manner. It is commonly used the population standard deviation and variance are unknown. As the sample size increases, the distribution becomes more normal.

$$t = \frac{\bar{X}_1 - \bar{X}_2}{SD_{pooled}\sqrt{\dfrac{1}{n_1} + \dfrac{1}{n_2}}}$$

Where:
$\bar{X}_1$ *and* $\bar{X}_2$ are the means of two independent sample sets. Each sample set also has a sample standard deviation ($SD_1\ and\ SD_2$).
n_1, n_2 are the number of measurements in each sample set.
SD_{pooled} is an estimate of the common SD.
Note: The numerator of the equation often shows: $- (u_1 - u_2)$ but if we assume that the population means are equal under the null hypothesis, then $(u_1 - u_2) = 0$.
Source: Principles of Biostatistics, Pagano, et al, 2nd edition

To continue with the previous example:
> Two groups of workers are selected from similar work areas in a lead acid battery manufacturing facility to compare the mean blood lead levels between the groups. The distribution is assumed normal and the variance assumed equal. The following results are obtained:
>
> Method 1: mean = 18.9 ug/dL, SD = 5.9 ug/dL, n = 9
> Method 2: mean = 11.9 ug/dL, SD = 6.3 ug/dL, n = 13

Test the hypothesis using a 2-sided test and a significance (α) of 0.05.

Step 1: State the null hypothesis: There is no difference between the true mean blood lead levels - $u_1 = u_2$

Step 2: Calculate the SD_{pooled}

$$SD_{pooled} = \sqrt{\frac{(n_1 - 1)SD_1{}^2 + (n_2 - 1)SD_2{}^2}{n_1 + n_2 - 2}}$$

$$SD_{pooled} = 6.1\ ug/dL$$

Step 3: Calculate the test statistic

$$t = \frac{\bar{X}_1 - \bar{X}_2}{SD_{pooled}\sqrt{\frac{1}{n_1} + \frac{1}{n_2}}}$$

$$t = \frac{18.9 - 11.9}{6.1 \text{ x }\sqrt{\frac{1}{9} + \frac{1}{13}}}$$

$$t = 2.63$$

Step 4: Refer to the t distribution table
        20 degrees of freedom $t_{20} = 2.63$ falls between 0.01 and 0.005

Percentiles of the t distribution

	Area in the Upper Tail					
Df	**0.10**	**0.05**	**0.025**	**0.01**	**0.005**	**0.0005**
16	1.337	1.746	2.120	2.583	2.921	4.015
17	1.333	1.740	2.110	2.567	2.898	3.965
18	1.330	1.734	2.101	2.552	2.878	3.922
19	1.328	1.729	2.093	2.539	2.861	3.833
20	1.325	1.725	2.086	**2.528**	**2.845**	3.850

This is a two-tailed test, accordingly the area is the sum of the area to the right of 2.63 and to the left of -2.63. This equates to a calculated probability that the two means are equal is between 0.01 and 0.02 (the sum of the areas for 0.01 and 0.005). This is the p-value.

Step 5: Compare the calculated p-value to the pre-determined level of significance $\alpha = 0.05$
        0.01 to 0.02 < 0.05, therefore reject the null hypothesis

One-Sided 95% Confidence Interval
When utilized with a mean the confidence interval produces a range of values in which the sample mean may fall. Confidence limits are either the upper confidence limit <u>OR</u> lower confidence limit and are the boundaries of the interval.

$$95\% \; Conf = \bar{X} \pm 1.645 \left(\frac{SD}{\sqrt{n}}\right)$$

Where:
$\bar{X}$ is the arithmetic mean.
95% $Conf$ is the one-sided 95% confidence limit. Again, either upper or lower.
1.645 is the constant value equivalent to 5% of the area for the standard deviation.
SD is the standard deviation.

Example:
Employees working in a lead acid battery manufacturing facility have blood tests monthly. The site nurse collects blood lead level information for analysis. The following results are obtained from the nurse:
$$Mean = 18.9 \; ug/dL, \; SD = 5.9 \; ug/dL, \; n = 100$$

Calculate the 95% lower confidence limit (LCL).

Step 1: Calculate the 95% lower confidence limit.

$$Lower \; Confidence \; Limit \; (LCL) = \bar{X} - 1.645 \left(\frac{SD}{\sqrt{n}}\right)$$

$$Lower \; Confidence \; Limit \; (LCL) = \left(18.9 \frac{\mu g}{dL}\right) - (1.645)\left(\frac{5.9 \frac{\mu g}{dL}}{\sqrt{100}}\right)$$

$$95\% \; LCL = 17.9 \; \frac{\mu g}{dL}$$

Source: Principles of Biostatistics, Pagano, et al, 2ⁿᵈ edition

Example:
Employees working in a lead acid battery manufacturing facility have blood tests monthly. The site nurse collects blood lead level information for analysis. The following results are obtained from the nurse:

$$\text{Mean} = 18.9 \text{ ug/dL}, \text{SD} = 5.9 \text{ ug/dL}, n = 100$$

Calculate the 95% upper confidence limit (UCL).

Step 1: Calculate the 95% upper confidence limit.

$$Upper\ Confidence\ Limit\ (UCL) = \bar{X} + 1.645 \left(\frac{SD}{\sqrt{n}}\right)$$

$$Upper\ Confidence\ Limit\ (UCL) = (18.9 \text{ ug/dL}) + (1.645)\left(\frac{5.9 \text{ ug/dL}}{\sqrt{100}}\right)$$

$$95\%\ UCL = 19.9 \text{ ug/dL}$$

Source: Principles of Biostatistics, Pagano, et al, 2nd

Two-sided 95% Confidence Interval

$$95\%\ Conf = \bar{X} \pm 1.965 \left(\frac{SD}{\sqrt{n}}\right)$$

Where:
$\bar{X}$ is the arithmetic mean.
95% _Conf_ is the one-sided 95% confidence limit. Again, either upper or lower.
1.645 is the constant value equivalent to 5% of the area for the standard deviation.
SD is the standard deviation.

The upper and lower confidence limits calculated in the previous examples form the confidence interval.
Source: Principles of Biostatistics, Pagano, et al, 2nd

Cumulative Error

Exposure measurement is a process that involves several steps. Each step has some random error. The error associated with each step contributes to the overall error. The overall error is termed cumulative error.

$$E_c = \sqrt{E_1^2 + E_2^2 + \cdots + E_n^2}$$

Where:

E_c is the cumulative error.

$E_1, E_2, \ldots E_n$ are the individual error or variability for each step. They may be expressed as coefficient of variation (CV), standard deviation, or variance.

To use coefficient of variation (CV), the equation is changed to:

$$CV_T = \sqrt{(CV_s)^2 + (CV_a)^2}$$

Where:

CV_T is the cumulative coefficient of variation.

CV_s the coefficient of variation of the sampling method, which is a derived value for specific sample methods.

CV_a is the coefficient of variation calculated for the specific analytical method.

Note: The coefficient of variation is the standard deviation/mean.

Example:

Calculate the total error for an exposure assessment. The literature lists CV, for the sample method as 3%, and the error for the analytical method as 12%.

Step 1: Calculate the cumulative error

$$CV_T = \sqrt{(CV_s)^2 + (CV_a)^2}$$

$$CV_T = \sqrt{[(0.03)^2 + (0.12)^2]}$$

$$CV_T = 0.123$$

Source: Industrial-Occupational Hygiene Calculations: A Professional Reference

The CV_T for many substances can be found in the NIOSH Occupational Exposure Sampling Strategy Manual. The Sampling and Analytical Error can then be calculated using:

$$SAE = 1.645(CV_T)$$

Lower Confidence Limit for Consecutive Samples

$$LCL = \frac{C_A}{PEL} - \frac{SAE \sqrt{T_1^2 C_1^2 + T_2^2 C_2^2 + \cdots + T_n^2 C_n^2}}{PEL(T_1 + T_2 + \cdots T_n)}$$

Where:
LCL is the lower confidence limit.
C_A is the time-weighted average (TWA) concentration for consecutive samples.
PEL is the Permissible Exposure Limit (PEL).
SAE is the Sampling and Analytical Error. It combines the errors associated with air flow, time, and laboratory analysis. It is utilized in decimal form.
$T_1, T_2, \ldots T_n$ are the individual sampling times for the consecutive samples in minutes.
$C_1, C_2, \ldots C_n$ are the measured concentrations.

Example:
A worker is assessed for exposure to tetrahydrofuran. Two consecutive air samples are required. Sample 1 is collected for 260 minutes, and the lab reports a concentration of 26.99 ppm. Sample 2 is taken immediately after the first sample for a period of 220 minutes, and the lab reports a concentration of 38.19 ppm. The CV_T for tetrahydrofuran is 0.06 according to NIOSH method S-78, and the PEL is 50ppm. The time-weighted average concentration of both samples is 34.64 ppm.

Calculate the Lower Confidence Limit for Consecutive Samples.

Step 1: Calculate the SAE

$$SAE = 1.645(CV_T)$$

$$SAE = 1.645(0.06)$$

$$SAE = 0.1$$

Step 2: Calculate the TWA for the sample period (C_A).

$$\frac{(260 \; x \; 26.99)+(220 \; x \; 38.19)}{480}$$

$$TWA = 32 \; ppm$$

Step 3: Calculate the Lower Confidence Limit for Consecutive Samples

$$LCL = \frac{C_A}{PEL} - \frac{SAE \sqrt{T_1^2 C_1^2 + T_2^2 C_2^2 + \cdots + T_n^2 C_n^2}}{PEL(T_1 + T_2 + \cdots T_n)}$$

$$LCL = \frac{32\ ppm}{50\text{ppm}} - \frac{0.10\sqrt{(26.99 ppm)^2(260\text{min})^2 + (38.19\text{ppm})^2(220\text{min})^2}}{50\text{ppm}(260 min + 220\text{min})}$$

$$LCL = 0.61$$

Since the LCL is less than the exposure, the exposure can be considered above the PEL with a 95% confidence level.

Source: Industrial-Occupational Hygiene Calculations: A Professional Reference

Rubric 5: Biostatistics and Epidemiology Questions

1. A study was conducted among a group of employees at Company XYZ to evaluate exposure to Acetone. The table represents eight Acetone exposure levels. The mean is 10.40 ppm.

Table: Acetone Exposure

Employee	Acetone Exposure (ppm)
1	15.9
2	20.6
3	11.9
4	4.1
5	2.5
6	7.5
7	12.3
8	8.4

Calculate the variance using the Acetone exposure table.

A) 12.5 ppm^2
B) 36.4 ppm^2
C) 58.0 ppm^2
D) 98.4 ppm^2

2. A study was conducted among a group of employees at Company XYZ to evaluate exposure to acetone. The table represents eight Acetone exposure levels for each employee. The mean is 10.40 ppm.

Table: Acetone Exposure

Employee	Acetone Exposure (ppm)
1	15.9
2	20.6
3	11.9
4	4.1
5	2.5
6	7.5
7	12.3
8	8.4

Calculate the standard deviation.

A) 1.14 ppm
B) 2.70 ppm
C) 5.43 ppm
D) 6.03 ppm

3. A set of 15 air samples was collected for measurement of exposure to total particulates. The results are 8.4 mg/m³, 10.5 mg/m³, 12.7 mg/m³, 18.9 mg/m³, 19.7 mg/m³, 20.6 mg/m³, 20.9 mg/m³, 21.1 mg/m³, 21.8 mg/m³, and 22.3 mg/m³. The data is presented in the table below.

Table: Geometric Mean (log form)

$X_i\ (mg/m^3)$	$Log\ X_i$
8.4	0.92
10.5	1.02
12.7	1.10
18.9	1.28
19.7	1.29
20.6	1.31
20.9	1.32
21.1	1.32
21.8	1.34
22.3	1.35
24.9	1.40
25.1	1.40
25.7	1.41
26.0	1.42
29.6	1.47
$\Sigma\ \log x_i = 19.35$	

Calculate the geometric mean (log form).

A) $19.50\ mg/m^3$
B) $24.67\ mg/m^3$
C) $34.33\ mg/m^3$
D) $56.89\ mg/m^3$

4. This use of the t-test is illustrated in a comparison of two analytical methods. Suppose we have two methods being used to analyze for toluene. An atmosphere of toluene vapor in air is generated, and 10 samples are collected with method 1, and 10 samples with method 2. The following results are obtained:

Method 1: mean = 75.51 ppm, SD = 3.15 ppm, n = 10
Method 2: mean = 74.23 ppm, SD = 2.98 ppm, n = 10

Perform the t-test and calculate the test statistic.
A) 0.40
B) 0.79
C) 0.93
D) 1.24

5. Personal grab samples were collected on an operator to monitor worker's exposure to ethanol (TLV 1,000 ppm). The following results were reported for 10 charcoal tubes each exposed for 20 minutes.

1220 ppm	850 ppm	1100 ppm	1450 ppm	970 ppm	980 ppm	550 ppm	1280 ppm	400 ppm	1300 ppm

$$\bar{x} = 1010 \ ppm$$
$$Sx = 335.76 \ ppm$$

Calculate the 95% upper confidence limit (UCL).

A) $1105.89 \ ppm$
B) $1126.66 \ ppm$
C) $1184.66 \ ppm$
D) $1289.43 \ ppm$

6. Two (2) air samples are taken to measure a worker's exposure to tetrahydrofuran. One sample is collected for 260 minutes and produces a concentration of 26.99 ppm. A second sample is taken immediately after the first sample for a period of 220 minutes, and a concentration of 38.19 ppm is obtained. The SAE for the measurement of tetrahydrofuran is 0.10, and the PEL is 50ppm. The time-weighted average concentration for both samples is 32.12ppm. Calculate the lower confidence limit for consecutive samples.

A) 0.60
B) 1.87
C) 2.61
D) 5.98

7. Which statement is true about the geometric mean?

A) It can be determined by a graphical technique using log-log graph paper
B) It is always dimensionless
C) It is the nth root of the product of n observations
D) It is always greater than the arithmetic mean

8. Which of the following situations could lead to an OSHA citation? (All confidence intervals at 95% confidence)

A) LCL > standard
B) UCL > standard
C) LCL < standard
D) UCL < standard
E) UCL < standard and LCL < standard

9. How do you calculate the coefficient of variation?

    A) The sample standard deviation divided by the sample mean
    B) The sample standard deviation multiplied by the sample mean
    C) The sample mean divided by the sample standard deviation
    D) The sample mean multiplied by the sample standard deviation

10. Choose the statement that best describes the mode.

    A) The value in a set of measurements that occurs most frequently; the maximum value of a continuous probability density function.
    B) The difference between the largest and smallest values in a measurement data set.
    C) A measure of central tendency, calculated as the sum of all values in a population divided by the number of values in the population.
    D) The exposure measurement that divides a set of measurements into two equal parts, with half less than and half greater than this value.

11. Choose the statement that best describes the Central Limit Theorem.

    A) Parameters used to make estimates about the exposure distribution and underlying population.
    B) A quantity that describes a statistical population (e.g., mean and standard deviation, geometric mean, geometric standard deviation).
    C) An important symmetric probability distribution characterized completely by two parameters: the mean and the standard deviation.
    D) The sampling distribution of the mean approaches a normal distribution as the sample size increases, regardless of the shape of the underlying population distribution.

12. Choose the statement that best describes the Decision statistic.

    A) The distribution of a random variable with the property such that the logarithms of its values are normally distributed.
    B) An estimate of the parameter selected to represent the acceptability of an exposure profile.
    C) Parameters used to make estimates about the exposure distribution and underlying population.
    D) A quantity that describes a statistical population (e.g., mean and standard deviation, geometric mean, geometric standard deviation).

13. Choose the statement that best describes the Normal distribution.

    A) A quantity that describes a statistical population (e.g., mean and standard deviation, geometric mean, geometric standard deviation).
    B) An estimate of the parameter selected to represent the acceptability of an exposure profile.
    C) The distribution of a random variable with the property such that the logarithms of its values are normally distributed.
    D) An important symmetric probability distribution characterized completely by two parameters: the mean and the standard deviation.

14. Choose the answer that best describes the main difference between incidence and prevalence?

    A) Incidence measures the disease frequency during a specific period of time, and prevalence measures the disease frequency at a given point in time.
    B) Prevalence measures the disease frequency during a specific period of time, and incidence measures the disease frequency at a given point in time.
    C) Incidence measures the disease frequency for the entire study population, and prevalence measures the disease frequency for a specified study population.
    D) Incidence measures the frequency of people with the disease, and prevalence measures the frequency of people without the disease.

15. Population of workers at Turner Construction on March 30, 2017 = 200,000
    Number of new active cases of musculoskeletal injuries occurring between January 1 and June 30, 2016 = 88
    Number of active musculoskeletal injuries in the Turner Construction register on June 30, 2017 = 12
    The incident rate of active cases of musculoskeletal injuries for the six (6) month period was:

    A) 34 per 100,000 population.
    B) 44 per 100,000 population.
    C) 78 per 100,000 population.
    D) 90 per 100,000 population.
    E) 130 per 100,000 population.

16. Population of workers at Turner Construction on March 30, 2016 = 200,000
    Number of new active cases of musculoskeletal injuries occurring between January 1 and June 30, 2017 = 88
    Number of active musculoskeletal injuries in the Turner Construction register on June 30, 2017 = 12
    The prevalence rate of musculoskeletal injuries as of June 30, 2017, was:

    A) 6 per 100,000 population.
    B) 12 per 100,000 population.
    C) 28 per 100,000 population.
    D) 73 per 100,000 population.

17. In order to assess how strongly related an exposure is to a disease, which would be the best health statistic?

    A) Incidence of the disease among the exposed.
    B) Attributable risk.
    C) Prevalence of the exposure.
    D) Relative Risk.
    E) Proportionate mortality.

18. In what type(s) of study designs is it possible to utilize the odds ratio?

    A) Case-control study.
    B) Randomized study.
    C) Cohort study and case-control study.
    D) Case-control study and randomized study.

19. Choose the study design that identifies a group of workers with a disease and examines their past work history for potential exposures?

    A) Cross-sectional study.
    B) Case-control retrospective study.
    C) Case-control prospective study.
    D) Mortality study.

20. Choose the study design that focuses on the prevalence of an outcome casual pathway at the time the survey is conducted.

    A) Randomized study.
    B) Case-control study.
    C) Cohort study.
    D) Cross-sectional study.

Rubric 5: Biostatistics and Epidemiology Answers

1. Answer B.

Explanation:

Table: Acetone Exposure

Employee	Acetone Exposure (ppm)
1	15.9
2	20.6
3	11.9
4	4.1
5	2.5
6	7.5
7	12.3
8	8.4

Table: Variance

Employee	Acetone Exposure (x_i)	$(\bar{x} - x_i)$	$(\bar{x} - x_i)^2$
1	15.9	-5.5	30.3
2	20.6	-10.2	104.0
3	11.9	-1.5	2.3
4	4.1	6.3	39.7
5	2.5	7.9	62.4
6	7.5	2.9	8.4
7	12.3	-1.9	3.6
8	8.4	2.0	4.0
Total	83.2	0	254.7

Calculate the variance:

$$s^2 = \frac{1}{(n-1)} \sum_{i=1}^{n} (\bar{x} - x_i)^2$$

$$s^2 = \frac{1}{(8-1)} \sum_{i=1}^{8} (10.40 - x_i)^2$$

$$s^2 = \frac{254.7}{7}$$

$$s^2 = 36.4 \; ppm^2$$

If you are using the TI 30X IIS, use the following calculation keystrokes:

Step 1 – Set to STAT Mode using the second function of DATA key

Step 2 – Select 1-VAR and Enter key

Step 3 – Press DATA key

Step 4 – Enter Data (X_1, down arrow key, FRQ, down arrow key; X_2, down arrow key, FRQ, down arrow key; … X_n, down arrow key, FRQ, down arrow key)

Step 5 – Press STATVAR key

Step 6 – Use arrow keys and select Sx

Step 7 – Square the value

2.   Answer D.
Explanation:

Employee	Acetone Exposure (ppm)
1	15.9
2	20.6
3	11.9
4	4.1
5	2.5
6	7.5
7	12.3
8	8.4

Table: Standard Deviation

Employee	Acetone Exposure (x_i)	$(\bar{x} - x_i)$	$(\bar{x} - x_i)^2$
1	15.9	-5.5	30.3
2	20.6	-10.2	104.0
3	11.9	-1.5	2.3
4	4.1	6.3	39.7
5	2.5	7.9	62.4
6	7.5	2.9	8.4
7	12.3	-1.9	3.6
8	8.4	2.0	4.0
Total	83.2	0	254.7

          Copyright©2019 SPAN International Training, LLC

Calculate the standard deviation:

$$SD = \sqrt{\frac{\Sigma(\bar{x} - x_i)^2}{n - 1}}$$

$$SD = \sqrt{\frac{\Sigma(10.40 - x_i)^2}{8 - 1}}$$

$$SD = \sqrt{\frac{254.7}{7}}$$

$$SD = 6.03 \; ppm$$

If you are using the TI 30X IIS, use the following calculation keystrokes:

Step 1 – Set to STAT Mode using the second function of DATA key

Step 2 – Select 1-VAR and Enter key

Step 3 – Press DATA key

Step 4 – Enter Data (X_1, down arrow key, FRQ, down arrow key; X_2, down arrow key, FRQ, down arrow key; … X_n, down arrow key, FRQ, down arrow key)

Step 5 – Press the STATVAR key

Step 6 – Use arrow keys and select Sx

3. Answer A.
   Explanation:

Geometric Mean (log form) table

X_i (mg/m^3)	Log X_i
8.4	0.92
10.5	1.02
12.7	1.10
18.9	1.28
19.7	1.29
20.6	1.31
20.9	1.32
21.1	1.32
21.8	1.34
22.3	1.35
24.9	1.40
25.1	1.40
25.7	1.41
26.0	1.42
29.6	1.47

$\sum \log x_i = 19.35$

Step 1: Calculate the sum of the base 10 logarithm of the values.

Table: Geometric Mean (log form)

X_i (mg/m^3)	Log X_i
8.4	0.92
10.5	1.02
12.7	1.10
18.9	1.28
19.7	1.29
20.6	1.31
20.9	1.32
21.1	1.32
21.8	1.34
22.3	1.35
24.9	1.40
25.1	1.40
25.7	1.41
26.0	1.42
29.6	1.47

$\sum \log x_i = 19.35$

Step 2: Calculate the geometric mean (log form)

$$GM = 10^{\frac{\Sigma(\log x)}{n}}$$

$$GM = 10^{19.35/15}$$
$$GM = 19.50 \, mg/m^3$$

4. Answer C.
   Explanation:

$$\text{Method 1: mean} = 75.51 \text{ ppm, SD} = 3.15 \text{ ppm, n} = 10$$
$$\text{Method 2: mean} = 74.23 \text{ ppm, SD} = 2.98 \text{ ppm, n} = 10$$

Step 1: Calculate the SD_{pooled}

$$SD_{pooled} = \sqrt{\frac{(n_1 - 1)SD_1{}^2 + (n_2 - 1)SD_2{}^2}{n_1 + n_2 - 2}}$$

$$SD_{pooled} = \sqrt{\frac{(9)(3.15)^2 + (9)(2.98)^2}{18}}$$

$$SD_{pooled} = 3.07$$

Step 2: Calculate the test statistic

$$t = \frac{\bar{X}_1 - \bar{X}_2}{SD_{pooled}\sqrt{\frac{1}{n_1} + \frac{1}{n_2}}}$$

$$t = \frac{75.51 - 74.23}{3.07\sqrt{\frac{1}{10} + \frac{1}{10}}}$$

$$t = 0.93$$

The value of t in a table of the t distribution shows the probability associated with a value of t = 0.93 with 18 degrees of freedom (n-2).
Source: Principles of Biostatistics, Pagano, et al, 2nd

t Distribution Table

Level of Confidence											
One-tail	0.50	0.25	0.20	0.15	0.10	0.05	0.025	0.01	0.005	0.001	0.0005
Two-tails	1.00	0.50	0.40	0.30	0.20	0.10	0.05	0.02	0.01	0.002	0.001
df											
1	0.0	1.0	1.376	1.936	3.078	6.314	12.71	31.82	63.66	318.31	636.62
2	0.0	.816	1.061	1.386	1.886	2.920	4.303	6.965	9.925	23.327	31.599
3	0.0	.765	.978	1.250	1.638	2.353	3.182	4.541	5.841	10.215	12.924
4	0.0	.741	.941	1.190	1.533	2.132	2.776	3.747	4.604	7.173	8.610
5	0.0	.727	.920	1.156	1.476	2.015	2.571	3.365	4.032	5.893	6.869
6	0.0	.718	.906	1.134	1.440	1.943	2.447	3.143	3.707	5.208	5.959
7	0.0	.711	.896	1.119	1.415	1.895	2.365	2.998	3.499	4.785	5.408
8	0.0	.706	.889	1.108	1.397	1.860	2.306	2.896	3.355	4.501	5.041
9	0.0	.703	.883	1.100	1.383	1.833	2.262	2.821	3.250	4.297	4.781
10	0.0	.700	.879	1.093	1.372	1.812	2.228	2.764	3.169	4.144	4.587
11	0.0	.697	.876	1.088	1.363	1.796	2.201	2.718	3.106	4.025	4.437
12	0.0	.695	.873	1.083	1.356	1.782	2.179	2.681	3.055	3.930	4.318
13	0.0	.694	.870	1.079	1.350	1.771	2.160	2.650	3.012	3.852	4.221
14	0.0	.692	.868	1.076	1.345	1.761	2.145	2.624	2.977	3.787	4.140
15	0.0	.691	.866	1.074	1.341	1.753	2.131	2.602	2.947	3.733	4.037
16	0.0	.690	.865	1.071	1.337	1.746	2.120	2.583	2.921	3.868	4.015
17	0.0	.689	.863	1.069	1.333	1.740	2.110	2.567	2.898	3.646	3.965
18	0.0	.688	**.862**	**1.067**	1.330	1.734	2.101	2.552	2.878	3.610	3.922
19	0.0	.688	.861	1.066	1.328	1.729	2.093	2.539	2.861	3.579	3.883
20	0.0	.687	.860	1.064	1.325	1.725	2.086	2.528	2.845	3.552	3.850
21	0.0	.686	.859	1.063	1.323	1.721	2.080	2.518	2.831	3.527	3.819
22	0.0	.686	.858	1.061	1.321	1.717	2.074	2.508	2.819	3.505	3.792
23	0.0	.685	.858	1.060	1.319	1.714	2.069	2.500	2.807	3.485	3.768
24	0.0	.685	.857	1.059	1.318	1.711	2.064	2.492	2.797	3.467	3.745
25	0.0	.684	.856	1.058	1.316	1.708	2.060	2.485	2.787	3.450	3.725
26	0.0	.684	.856	1.058	1.315	1.706	2.056	2.479	2.779	3.435	3.707
27	0.0	.684	.855	1.057	1.314	1.703	2.052	2.473	2.771	3.421	3.690
28	0.0	.683	.855	1.056	1.313	1.701	2.048	2.467	2.763	3.408	3.674
29	0.0	.683	.854	1.055	1.311	1.699	2.045	2.462	2.756	3.396	3.659
30	0.0	.683	.854	1.055	1.310	1.697	2.042	2.457	2.750	3.385	3.646
40	0.0	.681	.851	1.050	1.303	1.684	2.021	2.423	2.704	3.307	3.551
60	0.0	.679	.848	1.045	1.296	1.671	2.000	2.390	2.660	3.232	3.460
80	0.0	.678	.846	1.043	1.292	1.664	1.990	2.374	2.639	3.195	3.416
100	0.0	.677	.845	1.042	1.290	1.660	1.984	2.364	2.626	3.174	3.390
1000	0.0	.675	.842	1.037	1.282	1.646	1.962	2.330	2.581	3.098	3.300
Z	0.0	.674	.842	1.036	1.282	1.645	1.960	2.326	2.576	3.090	3.291
	0%	50%	60%	70%	80%	90%	95%	98%	99%	99.8%	99.9%

Confidence Level

5. Answer C.
    Explanation:

Calculate the 95% upper confidence limit.

$$Upper\ Confidence\ Limit\ (UCL) = \bar{X} + 1.645\left(\frac{SD}{\sqrt{n}}\right)$$

$$Upper\ Confidence\ Limit\ (UCL) = (1010\ ppm) + (1.645)\left(\frac{335.76\ ppm}{\sqrt{10}}\right)$$

$$95\%\ UCL = 1184.66\ ppm$$

Source: Industrial-Occupational Hygiene Calculations: A Professional Reference

6. Answer A.
    Explanation:

Calculate the Lower Confidence Limit for Consecutive Samples

$$LCL = \frac{C_A}{PEL} - \frac{SAE\ \sqrt{T_1^2 C_1^2 + T_2^2 C_2^2 + \cdots + T_n^2 C_n^2}}{PEL(T_1 + T_2 + \cdots T_n)}$$

$$LCL = \frac{32.12ppm}{50ppm} - \frac{0.10\sqrt{(26.99ppm)^2(260min)^2 + (38.19ppm)^2(220min)^2}}{50ppm(260min + 220min)}$$

LCL = 0.6

The exposure can be said to exceed the PEL at the 95% confidence level.
Source: Industrial-Occupational Hygiene Calculations: A Professional Reference

7. Answer C.
    Explanation: Geometric means can also be computed as the antilog of the average of the logarithms of the observations. The formula is shown below.

$$\bar{x}_g = \frac{1}{n}\sqrt{(x_1)(x_2)\ldots(x_n)} = antilog\left(\frac{logx_1 + logx_2 + \cdots logx_n}{n}\right)$$

Source: OSHA, Industrial Hygiene Manual

8. Answer A.
    Explanation: An OSHA citation could only be issued if the data indicates that a violation exists at the 95% confidence level. Therefore, the lower (95%) confidence limit of the TWA exposure estimate must exceed the standard.
    Source: OSHA, Industrial Hygiene Manual

9. Answer A.
Explanation:
Coefficient of Variation: The sample standard deviation divided by the sample mean (or population parameters). When comparing variations between distributions with different means, coefficients of variation should be used. Sometimes expressed as a percentage. Abbreviated CV.

$$CV = \frac{SD}{\bar{x}}$$

Source: A Strategy for Assessing and Managing Occupational Exposures 4th edition

10. Answer A.
Explanation:
Mode: The value in a set of measurements that occurs most frequently; the maximum value of a continuous probability density function. The mode of a lognormal distribution is less than the median, which is less than the mean. The mean, median, and mode of a normal distribution are equal.
Source: Industrial-Occupational Hygiene Calculations: A Professional Reference

11. Answer D.
Explanation:
Central Limit Theorem: The sampling distribution of the mean approaches a normal distribution as the sample size increases regardless of the shape of the underlying population distribution. *Source: Industrial-Occupational Hygiene Calculations: A Professional Reference*

12. Answer B.
Explanation:
Decision statistic: An estimate of the parameter selected to represent the acceptability of an exposure profile. For example, the 95th percentile is often used as the decision statistic when comparing an exposure profile to an OEL. *Source: Industrial-Occupational Hygiene Calculations: A Professional Reference*

13. Answer D.
Explanation:
Normal distribution: An important symmetric probability distribution characterized completely by two parameters: the mean and the standard deviation. It has its highest ordinate at the center and tails off to zero in both directions, forming a bell-shaped curve.
Source: Industrial-Occupational Hygiene Calculations: A Professional Reference

14. Answer A.

Explanation: <u>Incidence</u> is a measure of disease frequency. Incidence rates are designed to measure the rate at which people without a disease develop the disease during a specific period of time i.e. the number of new cases of a disease in a population over a period of time. Incidence only includes new cases or events and a specified period during which those events occurred. <u>Prevalence</u> measures the frequency of disease at a given point in time. It is defined as the number of affected persons present in the population at a specific time divided by the number of persons in the population at that time i.e. what proportion of the population is affected by the disease at that time. Prevalence can be viewed as a snapshot or a slice through the population at a point in time at which we determine who has the disease and who does not.
Source: Epidemiology 5th Edition, Leon Gordis

15. Answer B.

Explanation: Calculate the incident rate:

$$Incidence\ Rate = \frac{number\ of\ new\ cases\ of\ a\ disease\ in\ the\ time\ period}{population\ at\ risk\ of\ the\ disease\ in\ the\ time\ period}$$

$$Incidence\ Rate = \frac{88}{200,000} = 0.00044 \times 100,000 = 44\ per\ 100,000\ population$$

Source: Epidemiology 5th Edition, Leon Gordis

16. Answer A.

Explanation: Calculate the prevalence

$$Prevalence = \frac{total\ number\ of\ cases\ of\ a\ disease\ at\ a\ given\ time}{total\ popuation\ at\ risk\ at\ a\ given\ time}$$

$$Prevalence = \frac{12}{200,000} = 0.00006 \times 100,000 = 6.0\ per\ 100,000\ population$$

Source: Epidemiology 5th Edition, Leon Gordis

17. Answer D.

Explanation: Relative risk is defined as the ratio of the risk of disease in exposed individuals to the risk of disease in nonexposed individuals. Relative risk tells the assessor the size of the excess risk that the subject with exposure to a factor runs, compared with a subject without exposure to such a factor. Relative risk identifies subjects at a high risk of certain outcomes. The relative risk measures the strength of an association; thus, a high relative risk suggests etiology or causality. *Source: Epidemiology 5th Edition, Leon Gordis*

18. Answer C.

Explanation: In order to calculate a relative risk, we must have values for the incidence of the disease in the exposed and the incidence in the nonexposed, as can be obtained from a cohort study. In a case-control study, we do not know the incidence in the nonexposed population because we start with diseased people (cases) and nondiseased people (controls). In a case-control study, we cannot calculate the relative risk directly. The odds ratio can be obtained from either a cohort or a case-control study and can be used instead of the relative risk. Even though we cannot calculate a relative risk from a case-control study, under many conditions we can obtain a very good estimate of the relative risk from a case-control study using the odds ratio. *Source: Epidemiology 5th Edition, Leon Gordis*

19. Answer B.

Explanation: Identify a group of workers with disease and examine their work history for potential exposures. The study period must start at a time when all of the participants were free of the outcome of interest and when first exposure can be ascertained. Most occupational epidemiology studies are retrospective because they seek to answer the question "Did exposure to agent "X" increase the risk for disease "Y." *Source: Epidemiology 5th Edition, Leon Gordis*

20. Answer D.

Explanation: Select a group of workers irrespective of exposure or disease and measure over time. A cross-sectional study is focused on the prevalence of an outcome in a population that has a risk for exposure to a suspected agent in the outcome causal pathway at the time the survey is conducted. This type of design works well for acute illnesses and injuries, or when evaluating the effectiveness or success of an intervention. The advantages of a cross-sectional study include simple design and execution, ability to use intermediate conditions rather than the final outcome, and ability to compare the results to other populations with similar risk and exposures.

Rubric 6: Community Exposure

Workers and the general public are potentially exposed to hazardous agents in the breathing air, water, and on surfaces they contact. Air pollution as it relates to the field of industrial hygiene is covered in this section. Air pollution presents exposures to the entire population, including children, elderly and those with complicating conditions. The exposure period is continuous for a lifetime.

Important Terms and Concepts

Adiabatic – A process or condition for which no heat flows into or out of the system. The atmosphere is neutrally stable.
- Super Adiabatic – The temperature decrease with height is faster than the adiabatic lapse rate. This type of atmosphere is unstable with efficient mixing.

Air pollution – The presence of solids, liquids, or gasses in the outdoor air that are detrimental to humans, animals, and plants or property, as well as unreasonably interferes with the comfortable enjoyment of life and property. Exposure period = 168 hours/week for a lifetime.

Clean Air Act 1970 (amended 77 & 90) – Act that requires the EPA to set National Ambient Air Quality Standards (40 CFR part 50) for pollutants considered harmful to public health and the environment. The Clean Air Act identifies two types of national ambient air quality standards:
- *Primary standards* provide public health protection, including protecting the health of "sensitive" populations such as asthmatics, children, and the elderly.
- *Secondary standards* provide public welfare protection, including protection against decreased visibility and damage to animals, crops, vegetation, and buildings.

Greenhouse gas - Gas in the atmosphere that absorbs and emits radiation within the thermal infrared range. The primary greenhouse gases in Earth's atmosphere are water vapor, carbon dioxide, methane, nitrous oxide, and ozone.

Hazardous air pollutants (HAPs) - Hazardous air pollutants, also known as toxic air pollutants or air toxics, are pollutants that are known or suspected to cause cancer or other serious health effects, such as reproductive effects or birth defects, or adverse environmental effects.

Isokinetic samples – Method required for particulate sampling in stack stream. The sample stream is at the same velocity as the exhaust stream.

Lapse rate – The decrease in temperature associated with the increase in elevation.

Man-made pollution – Fuel and energy production, fuel utilization, and industrial processes.

National Ambient Air Quality Standards (NAAQs) - The EPA has set National Ambient Air Quality Standards for six principal (criteria) pollutants:

- Ozone
- Carbon Monoxide
- Sulfur Dioxide
- Particulate Matter – PM_{10} and $PM_{2.5}$
- Lead
- Nitrogen Dioxide

Natural pollution sources – Volcanoes, fires, bacterial action (methane), plants.

Primary pollutants – Originate from the source. For example, NO_2 emitted from the industrial stack.

Secondary pollutants – Arise from atmospheric reactions and transformations. For example, photochemical smog = $O_3 + NO_x + HC + UV_{light}$.

Smog - A type of air pollutant. The word "smog" was coined in the early 20th century as a portmanteau of the words smoke and fog to refer to smoky fog.

5 Types of Exhaust Plumes

Exhaust plumes are dependent on atmospheric conditions such as temperature and pressure. These images show the 5 types of plumes.

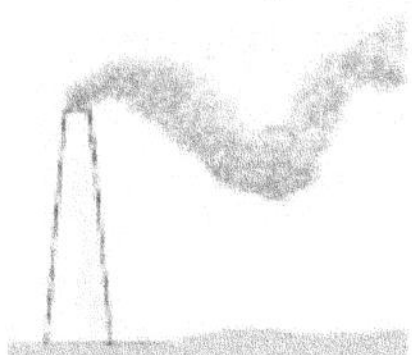 **Looping plume** – Unstable atmosphere. Associated with convective heating (sun).

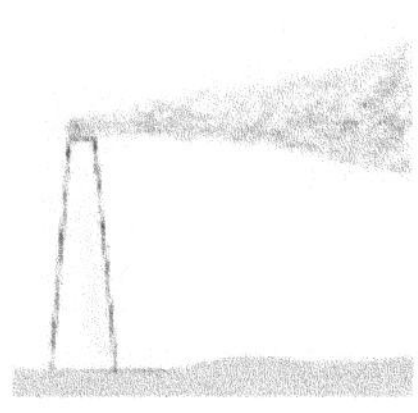 **Coning plume** – Neutral or stable atmosphere. Cloud cover decreases convection.

 **Fanning plume** – Inversion from the ground to above the plume. Most likely at night.

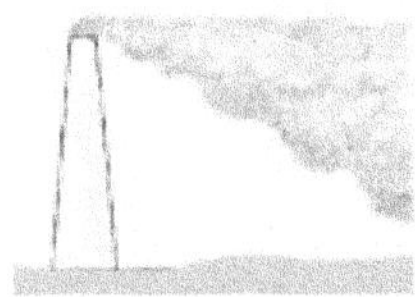 **Fumigating plume** – Inversion above the plume and unstable below. Usually in the morning following a period of significant stability.

 **Lofting plume** – Inversion below plume and unstable above. Late afternoon or early evenings. Conditions are opposite of fumigation.

Air Pollution Control Equipment

TYPE	OPERATION OVERVIEW	COMMENTS
Gravity Settling Device	Chamber with low velocity that allows particles to settle. The length of the chamber is important for design and function.	Chip trap. Old technology. Low efficiency.
Cyclone collector – Centrifugal separator	Air flow introduced into conical collector. Particles impact the wall and fall to the bottom for collection and air exhausts out the top.	Wet or dry, single or multi-cones. Dry inertial types are effective for particles > 10 µm. Both efficiency and pressure drop with decreasing flow rate.
Filter Devices	*Bag house* – air flows across series of bags and particles collect on surface. *Sand bed* – air ascends or water descends through large bed of sand and particles are collected in the sand. *Filter collection* – air stream or liquid passes through appropriate media.	*Bag house* – 99.8% efficient for particles > 0.5 µm diameter. Requires shaker system and regular maintenance. *Sand bed filter* – Up to 99.97% efficient. *Filters* – Up to 99.9% efficient. Requires regular maintenance.
Electrostatic Precipitator	High voltage produces a charge that attracts particles to the positive or negative electrode as air passes through the chamber. The charge is removed and particles fall into collection bins.	Efficiency increases with length. Significant energy consumption. Low pressure drop.
Wet Scrubbers	*Static* – air forced through water in a container. *Inertial* – wet cyclone. *Countercurrent* – air moves up as liquid moves down. *Water spray* – water is sprayed in opposite direction of air.	Venturi has major maintenance challenges. Wet cyclone -Up to 90% efficient for particles > 5 µm. Drawbacks: sludge accumulation, not good for cold climates.
Adsorbent	Air stream passes through media - typically activated charcoal.	Not effective for high temperature operations.
Incinerator	Air stream passes through chamber that is $> 1000°F$ burning combustible gasses and particles.	Air stream may then pass onto absorption media. Used for VOCs primarily.
Catalytic converter	Air stream passes through catalyst (platinum) resulting in a reaction with O_2.	Expensive catalyst.

Air Pollution Models

These models are required in the regulatory control of air quality. The models are:

- **Box model** – Based on an assumed box of air over a city that is perfectly mixed (homogeneous).
- **Gridded model** – The model is based on the Urban Air-shed Model and is used for ozone modeling.
- **Source-oriented model** – Used to provide an estimate of airborne concentrations of pollutants downwind from the source based on estimates of emission rates and meteorological conditions.

Rubric 6: Community Exposure Questions

1. The following pollution controls operate by driving particulates to a wall or surface where they agglomerate into sand-like masses for collection and disposal:

    A) Gravity settling chambers, cyclones, and electrostatic precipitators.
    B) Gravity settling chambers, depth filters, surface filters.
    C) Cyclones, surface filters, venturi scrubber.
    D) Depth filter, surface filter, venturi scrubber.

2. The Clean Air Act identifies two types of ambient air quality standards. One provides public health protection, including protection for the health of sensitive individuals, while the other provides public welfare protection, including protection against decreased visibility and damage to animals, crops, vegetation, and buildings. The two standards are:

    A) Mandatory, voluntary.
    B) Criteria, non-criteria.
    C) Human health, environmental health.
    D) Primary, secondary.

3. During stack sampling for particles, what is the effect on the results if the sample flow velocity is greater than the stack flow velocity?

    A) The measured concentration is greater than the actual concentration.
    B) The measured concentration is less than the actual concentration.
    C) The measured concentration is proportional to the square of the actual concentration.
    D) The measured concentration is equal to the actual concentration.

4. Choose the answer that is the primary concern when dealing with air pollution.
    A) Human health.
    B) Visibility.
    C) Property damage.
    D) Threats to global climate.

5. Select a common method of emission control for a gaseous exhaust stream?
    A) Filtration.
    B) Masking.
    C) Concentration.
    D) Scrubbing/Liquid Absorption.

6. A "lapse rate" is the decrease in ___________ with an increase in ___________.
    A) Temperature; Elevation.
    B) Elevation; Temperature.
    C) Time; Temperature.
    D) Temperature; Time.

7. In terms of "isokinetic" sampling for particles:

   A) If the probe velocity is more than the stack velocity, then the measured concentration will be higher than the true stack concentration.
   B) If the probe velocity is more than the stack velocity, then the measured concentration will be lower than the true stack concentration.
   C) The probe velocity should be more than the stack velocity.
   D) The probe velocity should be less than the stack velocity.

8. An average flow rate of a stack is 1000 CFM and has an average SO_2 concentration of 1000 ppm. What is the mass emission rate of SO_2 in pounds per hour?

   A) 1 to 2 lb/hr.
   B) 2 to 4 lb/hr.
   C) 4 to 6 lb/hr.
   D) Greater than 6 lb/hr.

9. What is the overall efficiency of three series particulate collectors with efficiencies 75, 80, and 90%?

   A) 99.5%.
   B) 95%.
   C) 90%.
   D) 80%.

10. Control equipment is vital when dealing with pollutants. Four factors need to be identified when understanding if an air cleaner is needed. Three of the four factors are toxicity of the material, amount of material, and value of material. What is the fourth factor?

    A) Mass of material.
    B) Carcinogenicity of material.
    C) Government regulations.
    D) Local regulations.

11. Applying the chemiluminescent principal shall generate a measurement of:

    A) A wide variety of organic compounds.
    B) Trace metals.
    C) Oxides of sulfur.
    D) NO and ozone.

12. What characterizes electrostatic precipitators?

    A) Increased efficiency as length of passage through precipitator increases.
    B) High efficiency, low cost, and high pressure drop.
    C) High efficiency for dry particles, not useful for wet particles.
    D) Increasing efficiency and pressure drop with time of operation.

13. A stack is emitting an air pollutant. Maximum downwind ground level pollutant concentrations will normally:

    A) Decrease proportionally to the square of the effective plume height.
    B) Be independent of wind velocity.
    C) Be independent of temperature of stack effluent at stack outlet.
    D) Increase with the square of the pollutant emission rate.

14. The diagram illustrates what type of plume?

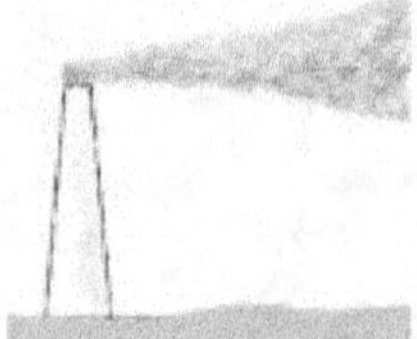

    A) Fanning.
    B) Fumigating.
    C) Looping.
    D) Coning.

15. The diagram illustrates what type of plume?

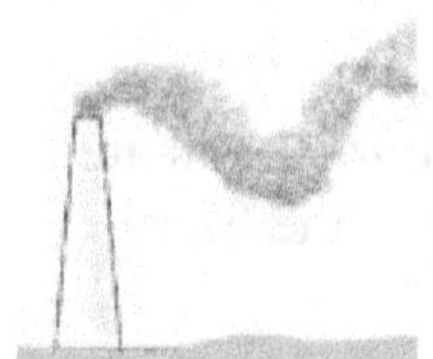

    A) Fanning.
    B) Fumigating.
    C) Looping.
    D) Coning.

16. An environmental engineer is testing your pollution control knowledge in a staff meeting. The site is reviewing a new process that will emit ammonia. Select the most appropriate air cleaning device for ammonia.

    A) Electrostatic precipitator.
    B) Sand filter bed.
    C) Absorber.
    D) It is not possible to remove the ammonia from the air stream.

17. There is a statement in environmental work: "Dilution is the solution to pollution." Select the best example of a dilution method.

   A) Tall stack.
   B) Venturi scrubber.
   C) HEPA filter.
   D) Electrostatic precipitator.

18. You have been asked to assist a church pew manufacturer in the Ozark Mountains to select a device for wood dust particle control. Select the most appropriate device.

   A) Venturi.
   B) Cyclone.
   C) Electrostatic precipitator.
   D) HEPA filter.

19. According to the US EPA, tropospheric ozone is formed when sunlight reacts with the following in the atmosphere.

   A) Oxides of nitrogen, volatile organic compounds.
   B) Oxides of sulfur, oxides of nitrogen.
   C) Chlorine, fluorine.
   D) Carbon monoxide, carbon dioxide, carbon disulfide.

20. What type of plume displays inversion below plume and unstable above and occurs late afternoon or early evenings?

   A) Looping.
   B) Fanning.
   C) Lofting.
   D) Reclining.

Rubric 6: Community Exposure Answers

1. Answer A.
   Explanation: These are different devices; however, each produces a layer of sand like particles that must be removed. *Source: Air Pollution Control Engineering, 2nd Edition*

2. Answer D.
   Explanation: The Clean Air Act identifies two types of national ambient air, including protecting the health of "sensitive" populations such as asthmatics, children, and the elderly. ***Secondary standards*** provide public welfare protection, including protection against decreased visibility and damage to animals, crops, vegetation, and buildings. *Source: US EPA 2016*

3. Answer B.
   Explanation: If sampling velocity is greater than the stack flow, then large particles will not be properly sampled and the measured result will be lower than the actual concentration. If sampling velocity is less than the stack flow, then the higher inertia of large particles will result in oversampling, and the measured result will be higher than the actual concentration. FIH 6th ed.

4. Answer A.
   Explanation: Industrial hygiene is concerned almost exclusively with human health; air pollution is primarily concerned with human health, but also concerned with visibility, property damage and threats to the global climate. *Source: Air Pollution Control Engineering, 2nd Edition*

5. Answer D.
   Explanation: The most common method of gas stream control is scrubbing/liquid absorption. *Source: Modern Industrial Hygiene, Volume 3*

6. Answer A.
   Explanation: A lapse rate is the decrease in temperature with an increase in elevation. The average value for the USA is 3.5°F/1000ft. = 6.5°C C/km. Note the sign; it is defined to be a positive number, thus indicating the temperature decreases as elevation increases. In an inversion, the lapse rate is negative, thus indicating that the temperature increases as elevation increases. *Source: Air Pollution Control Engineering, 2nd Edition*

7. Answer B.
   Explanation: If sampling velocity is greater than the stack flow, then large particles will not be properly sampled and the measured result will be lower than the actual concentration. If sampling velocity is less than the stack flow, then the higher inertia of large particles will result in oversampling, and the measured result will be higher than the actual concentration. FIH 6th ed.

---

8. Answer D.
   Explanation:
   Step 1: Calculate the mass of emission assuming Normal Temperature and Pressure

   $$MW \text{ of } SO_2 = 32 + 2(16) = 64$$
   $$mg/m^3 = \frac{ppm \; x \; mw}{24.45}$$

   $$mg/m^3 = \frac{1000(64)}{24.45} = 2{,}617 \; mg/m^3$$

   Step 2: Convert mg/m^3 to $pounds/m^3$

   $$2{,}617 \; mg/m^3 \; x \; \frac{g}{1000 \; mg} \; x \; \frac{lb}{454 \; g} = 0.006 \; lb/m^3$$

   Step 3: Convert CFM to m^3/hr

   $$\frac{1000 \; ft^3}{min} \; x \; \frac{m^3}{35.3 \; ft^3} \; x \; \frac{60 \; min}{hr} = 1700 \; m^3/hr$$

   Step 4: Calculate the pounds per hour

   $$\frac{0.006 \; lb}{m^3} \; x \; \frac{1700 \; m^3}{hr} = 10 \; lb/hr$$

   Single calculation method:

   $$\frac{1000 \; FT^3}{min} \; x \; \frac{60 \; min}{hr} \; x \; \frac{2{,}617 \; mg}{m^3} \; x \; \frac{m^3}{35.3 \; FT^3} \; x \; \frac{lb}{454 \; gm} \; x \; \frac{gm}{1000 \; mg} = 9.8 \; lb/hr$$

Note: Difference due to rounding.

9. Answer A.
   Explanation:
   Table: Efficiency of Three Series Particulate Collector

Collector Efficiency (%)	Filtration Calculation	Outcome (%)
75	0.75 x 1 = 0.75 1.0 - 0.75 = 0.25	25
80	0.80 x 0.25 = 0.20 0.25 - 0.20 = 0.05	5
90	0.90 x 0.05 = 0.045 0.05 - 0.045 = 0.005	0.5
Solve: 100% - 0.5% = 99.5%		

10. Answer C.
    Explanation: Four factors are taken into account to figure out if an air cleaner is needed when controlling for pollutants. The four factors are toxicity of the material, amount of material, value of material, and government regulations. *Source: Industrial Hygiene Reference and Study Guide, 3rd edition*

11. Answer D.

   Explanation: Concentrations of nitrogen dioxide (NO_2) in ambient air are determined indirectly by photometrically measuring the light intensity, at wavelengths greater than 600 nm, resulting from the chemiluminescent reaction of nitric oxide (NO) with ozone (O_3). NO_2 is first quantitatively reduced to NO by a converter. The NO, which commonly exists in association with NO_2, passes through the converter unchanged, thus resulting in a total nitrogen oxides (NO_X) concentration of NO plus NO_2. A portion of the ambient air is also reacted with O_3 without having passed through the converter, and the NO concentration is measured. This value is subtracted from the NO_X concentration yielding the concentration of NO_2. *Source: Reference Method for the Determination of Nitrogen Dioxide in the Atmosphere (Chemiluminscence)*

12. Answer A.

   Explanation: As particles are collected on the proximal collectors they become less effective; however, if more collectors follow then more particles will be collected. A longer path allows for more collectors. *Source: Air Pollution Control Engineering, 2nd Edition*

13. Answer A.

   Explanation: Greater plume height results in greater dilution of the plume at ground level. *Source: Air Pollution Control Engineering, 2nd Edition*

14. Answer D.

   Explanation: Coning plumes occur when there is a neutral or stable condition. *Source: Industrial Hygiene Reference and Study Guide. 3rd Edition*

15. Answer C.

   Explanation: Looping plumes occur when there are unstable conditions. *Source: Industrial Hygiene Reference and Study Guide. 3rd Edition*

16. Answer C.

   Explanation: The electrostatic precipitator and sand filter are better choices for particulates. Absorbers are used for removing gasses from air streams. *Source: Air Pollution Control Engineering. 2nd Edition*

17. Answer A.

   Explanation: A stack without any filtration or treatment is a method to put the emissions high enough to prevent adverse effects. This is based on the premises of mixing and dilution.

18. Answer B.

   Explanation: The cyclone is frequently used in wood shops to remove dust particles from the air. The venturi is a high maintenance device that is effective for small particles. Precipitators are energy intense and better suited for fine particles. HEPA filters are best suited for small particles and would be subject to frequent overloading and maintenance issues. *Source: Industrial Hygiene Reference and Study Guide. 3ʳᵈ Edition*

19. Answer A.
    Explanation: $NO_X + VOC \rightarrow O_3$
    Source: US EPA

20. Answer C.
    Explanation: A lofting plume occurs when there is an inversion below plume and unstable above. Late afternoon or early evenings. *Source: Industrial Hygiene Reference and Study Guide. 3ʳᵈ Edition*

Rubric 7: Engineering Controls and Ventilation

Important Terms and Concepts

Aerosol- Small solid or liquid particles suspended in air with diameters ranging from less than 0.01 μm to 100 μm.

Air Cleaner- A device designed to remove atmospheric contaminants, such as dusts, gases, vapors, fumes, and smokes.

Air Handling Unit (AHU)- The ventilation equipment in heating and air conditioning systems.

Anemometer- A device to measure air speed.

ASHRAE- American Society of Heating, Refrigeration, and Air Conditioning Engineers.

Barometer- A device for measuring atmospheric pressure using a working fluid, usually mercury. A long glass tube, closed at one end, evacuated, filled with mercury and inverted in a container of mercury. The height of the column of mercury is a measure of atmospheric pressure.

Brake Horsepower (BHP)- Horsepower (HP) required to drive a fan, taking into account the energy losses of fan. It is only determined by testing the fan.

Capture Velocity- Air velocity at any point in front of the hood needed to overcome opposing air currents and to capture the contaminated air by causing it to flow into the exhaust hood.

Conservation of Mass- In all ordinary chemical changes, the total mass of the reactants is always equal to the total mass of the products.

Coefficient of Entry- The actual rate of flow caused by a given hood static pressure compared to the theoretical flow that would result if the static pressure could be converted to velocity pressure with 100 percent efficiency. It is the ratio of actual to theoretical flow. C_e represents the percentage of flow into a given hood based on the static pressure of the given branch.

Density Correction Factor (d)- A factor to correct or convert air density at any temperature and pressure to equivalent conditions at ACGIH ventilation defined standard conditions (STP) and back as needed.

Duct- A conduit used for conveying air at low pressures.

Duct velocity- Air velocity through the duct cross section.

Dust- Small solid particles created by breaking larger solids.

Emission Factor- The statistical average of the amount of a specific pollutant emitted from each type of polluting source in relation to the quantity of material handled, processed, or burned.

Entry loss- The loss in pressure caused by air flowing into a duct or hood expressed as inches w.g..

Exhaust ventilation- The removal of air, typically by mechanical means, from a space. The flow of air between two points is because of a pressure difference between the two points. The flow is from the high-pressure to the low-pressure zone.

Face velocity- Average air velocity into the exhaust system measured at the opening into the hood or booth.

Fan laws- Statements and equations that describe the relationship between fan volume, pressure, brake horsepower, size, and rotating speed (RPM).

Fumes- Small solid particles formed by the condensation of vapors generated by heating, melting, and vaporization of solids.

Gasses- Formless liquids that tend to uniformly occupy their container space.

General Ventilation- Ventilation method consisting of either natural or mechanically induced fresh air movements to mix with and dilute contaminants in the workplace air. Not recommended to control toxic contaminants.

Hood- An enclosure, part of a local exhaust system.

Hood Entry Loss- The pressure loss from turbulence and friction as air enters the ventilation system.

Hood, slot - A hood consisting of a narrow slot that lead into a plenum under suction to distribute air velocity along the length of the slot.

Hood Static Pressure- The (suction) static pressure in a duct near a hood representing the suction that is available to draw air into the hood.

Local Exhaust Ventilation- A ventilation system that captures and removes contaminants at the point of origin before they escape into the workroom air.

Manometer- A device that measures pressure difference. Usually a U-shaped glass tube containing water or mercury.

Makeup Air- Clean, tempered outdoor air supplied to replace air removed by exhaust ventilation or by industrial processes.

Mists- Droplets of materials that are a liquid at normal temperature and pressure.

Mixing Factor- A dimensionless quantity that is used to adjust the volume of air moving in a space to account for air distribution.

Pitot Tube- A device consisting of two concentric tubes: one measures the total or impact pressure existing in the airstream, the other measures the static pressure. When the annular space between the tubes and the interior of the center tube are connected across a pressure-measuring device, the pressure difference automatically nullifies the static pressure, and the output is velocity pressure.

Plenum- Pressure-equalizing chamber.

Smoke- Aerosol suspension originating from combustion or sublimation.

Standard Air- Dry air at 70 degrees Fahrenheit and 29.92 inches of mercury. Equivalent to $\frac{0.075\ lb}{ft^3}$.

Static Pressure (SP)- The potential pressure exerted in all directions by a fluid (air) at rest. For a fluid in motion, it is measured at a right angle to the direction of flow. It shows the tendency to burst or collapse the pipe. When added to velocity pressure, it gives total pressure.

Static pressure regain- The increase in static pressure in a system as air velocity decreases and velocity pressure is converted into static pressure according to Bernoulli's theorem.

Substitution- Substituting a less hazardous material, equipment, or process for a more hazardous one (e.g., use of soap and water in place of solvents, use of automated equipment in place of manually operated equipment).

Total Pressure (TP)- The algebraic sum of the velocity pressure and the static pressure.

Traverse- A pitot traverse involves measuring the velocity at a number of points across the duct area. The velocity distribution is not uniform within the duct. A pitot tube is usually used for the traverse, but any velometer with a narrow probe sensor may also be used.

Vapor- Gaseous form of a substance that is normally a solid or liquid.

Velocity Pressure- Pressure exerted by air in motion. It has a positive value in the direction of air flow and is determined by subtracting static pressure from the total pressure.

Velometer- A device for measuring air velocity.

Ventilation, dilution- Airflow designed to dilute contaminants to acceptable levels. Also called general ventilation.

Sources: Fundamentals of Industrial Hygiene 5th Edition & The Occupational Environment: Its Evaluation, Control and Management, 3rd Edition

Ventilation Calculations

Volumetric Flow Rate Through a Duct

$$Q = VA$$

Where:
Q is the volumetric flow rate, expressed as actual cubic feet per minute (CFM)
V is the velocity of the moving gas (air), expressed as feet per minute (fpm)
A is the cross-sectional area of the duct or hood, expressed as square feet (ft^2)
Use:
To predict the volumetric flow rate.

Example:
Calculate the average duct velocity in a 6-inch diameter; round duct if the volumetric flow rate is 1500 cfm.

$$Q = VA \quad \text{or} \quad V = \frac{Q}{A}$$

$$Q = 1500 \text{ cfm}$$
$$A = \text{cross sectional area}$$

Step 1: Find the Area

$$A = \pi r^2$$

$$A = \pi \, (0.0625 \, ft^2)$$

$$A = 0.196 \, ft^2$$

Step 2: Solve for V

$$V = \frac{1,500 \, CFM}{0.196 \, ft^2}$$

$$V = 7653.1 \, fpm$$

Duct Area and Velocity Relationship

$$V_1 A_1 = V_2 A_2$$

Where:
V is the velocity of the moving gas (air), expressed as feet per minute (fpm)
A is the cross-sectional area of the duct or opening, expressed as square feet (ft^2)

Use: To describe the principal of the conservation of mass in regards to the flow of air in industrial ventilation systems

Example:
What is the velocity of air flowing through a 10-inch diameter duct if the velocity through a 5-inch diameter duct is 2000 fpm?

$$V_1 A_1 = V_2 A_2$$

Step 1: Solve for A_1

$$A_1 = \pi \left(\frac{5}{12}\right)^2$$

$$A_1 = 0.54 ft^2$$

Step 2: Solve for A_2

$$A_2 = \pi \left(\frac{2.5}{12}\right)^2$$

$$A_2 = 0.14 ft^2$$

Step 3: Solve for V_1

$$V_1 = \frac{V_2 A_2}{A_1}$$

$$V_1 = \frac{2000\ fpm \times 0.14 ft^2}{0.54 ft^2}$$

$$V_1 = 518\ fpm$$

Simplified Fan Laws

$$Q_2 = Q_1 \left(\frac{Size_2}{Size_1}\right)^3 \left(\frac{RPM_2}{RPM_1}\right)$$

$$P_2 = P_1 \left(\frac{Size_2}{Size_1}\right)^2 \left(\frac{RPM_2}{RPM_1}\right)^2$$

$$PWR_2 = PWR_1 \left(\frac{Size_2}{Size_1}\right)^5 \left(\frac{RPM_2}{RPM_1}\right)^3$$

Where:
Q is the volumetric flow rate expressed as actual cubic feet per minute (CFM)
P is the pressure typically expressed as inches on water gauge (w.g.)
PWR is power expressed as horse power (hp)
Size is the size of the fan in any consistent unit

Use: Assist with determining the effect of changing one of the above parameters within a specific group of fans on the other parameters.

Note: Flow varies directly with RPM, Pressure varies as the square of RPM, and power varies as the cube of RPM.

Example: The effect of changing rotation rate (RPM)

A fan fly wheel was changed by maintenance, increasing the fan rotation rate from 200 to 300 RPM. The original volumetric flow was 1000 CFM. What is the new volumetric flow?

$$Q_2 = Q_1 \left(\frac{Size_2}{Size_1}\right)^3 \left(\frac{RPM_2}{RPM_1}\right)$$

Step 1: Solve for Q_2

$$Q_2 = 1,000 \; CFM \left(\frac{1}{1}\right)^3 \left(\frac{300 \; RPM}{200 \; RPM}\right)$$

Note: The size did not change, so it is $\frac{1}{1}$

$$Q_2 = 1,500 \; CFM$$

Total Pressure of Air in a Duct

$$TP = VP + SP$$

Where:

TP is the total pressure, which is the sum of the static pressure and the velocity pressure, expressed as inches of water gauge (w.g.)

VP is the velocity pressure, which is the kinetic pressure in the direction of flow, expressed as inches of water gauge (w.g.)

SP is the static pressure, which is the potential pressure exerted in all directions by a fluid at rest, expressed as inches of water gauge (w.g.)

Use:

To describe the relationship between total pressure, velocity pressure and static pressure within a duct.

Example:

A manometer on the suction side of a fan is reading 0.56 inches w.g. velocity pressure and -1.1 inches w.g. static pressure. What is the total pressure on the suction side of the fan?

$$TP = VP + SP$$

$$VP = 0.56 \text{ inches w.g.}$$
$$SP = -1.1 \text{ inches w.g.}$$

Step 1: Solve for TP

$$TP = VP + SP$$

$$TP = 0.56 \; inches \; w.g. + (-1.1 \; inches \; w.g.)$$

$$TP = -0.54 \; inches \; w.g.$$

Fan Static Pressure

$$FSP = SP_{out} - SP_{in} - VP_{in}$$

Where:

FSP is fan static pressure that is the total pressure diminished by the fan velocity pressure, expressed as inches of water gauge (w.g.)

VP_{in} is the velocity pressure, which is the kinetic pressure in the direction of flow in, expressed as inches of water gauge (w.g.)

$SP_{in,\ out}$ is the static pressure, which is the potential pressure at the inlet and outlet of the fan, expressed as inches of water gauge (w.g.)

Use: To determine the relationship between the fan static pressure (FSP), and the system (duct) inlet and outlet static pressures (SP), and the inlet velocity pressure (VP).

Example:

A manometer took several readings on a fan's inlet and outlet sides. Calculate the fan static pressure (FSP) if the static pressure on the outlet side of the fan is 0.8 inches w.g., static pressure on the inlet side of the fan is 3.8 inches w.g., and the velocity pressure is 1.0 inches w.g.

$$FSP = SP_{out} - SP_{in} - VP_{in}$$

$$Sp_{out} = 0.8 \ inches \ w.\,g.$$
$$SP_{in} = 3.8 \ inches \ w.\,g.$$
$$VP_{in} = 1.0 \ inches \ w.\,g.$$

Step 1: Solve for FSP

$$FSP = SP_{out} - SP_{in} - VP_{in}$$

$$FSP = 0.8 \ inches \ w.\,g. -(-3.8 \ inches \ w.\,g.) - \ 1.0 \ inches \ w.\,g.$$

$$FSP = 3.6 \ inches \ w.\,g.$$

Fan Total Pressure

$$FTP = SP_{out} - SP_{in}$$

Where:

FTP is the fan total pressure or the fan total static pressure drop, expressed as inches of water gauge (w.g.)

SP_{out} is the static pressure (SP) on the outlet side of the fan, expressed as inches of water gauge (w.g.)

SP_{in} is the static pressure (SP) on the inlet side of the fan, expressed as inches of water gauge (w.g.)

Use: To describe all energy requirements for moving air through the ventilation system. It is calculated by adding the absolute values of the average total pressures found from the fan.

Example:

The inlet and outlet conditions at a fan include the following:

SP_{out} = 0.20 inches w.g.
SP_{in} = -0.80 inches w.g.
VP_{in} = VP_{out} = 0.25 inches w.g.

$$FTP = SP_{out} - SP_{in}$$

$$SP_{out} = 0.20 \ inches \ w.g.$$
$$SP_{in} = -0.80 \ inches \ w.g.$$

Step 1: Solve for FTP

$$FTP = 0.20 \ inches \ w.g. - (-0.80 \ inches \ w.g)$$

$$FTP = 1.00 \ inch \ w.g.$$

Velocity and Velocity Pressure Relationship

$$V = 4005\sqrt{VP}$$

Where:

V is the velocity of the moving gas (air), expressed as feet per minute (fpm)

VP is the velocity pressure, which is the kinetic pressure in the direction of flow, expressed as inches of water gauge (w.g.)

Use: To describe the relationship between the velocity (V), and velocity pressure (VP), of air moving within a duct.

Note: Standard air has a density of $0.075\frac{lbm}{ft^3}$. The constant 4005 is derived from the equation below.

$$V = 1096\sqrt{\frac{VP}{0.075\frac{lbm}{ft^2}}}$$

Example:

Calculate the velocity of air flowing through a 10-inch diameter duct if the velocity pressure in the duct is 3.4 inches w.g.

$$V = 4005\sqrt{VP}$$

$$VP = 3.4 \; inches \; w.\,g.$$

Step 1: Solve for V

$$V = 4005\sqrt{3.4}$$

$$V = 7385 \; fpm$$

Velocity and Velocity Pressure Relationship

$$V = 1096 \sqrt{\frac{VP}{\rho}}$$

Where:

V is the velocity of the moving gas (air), expressed as feet per minute (fpm)

VP is the velocity pressure, which is the kinetic pressure in the direction of flow, expressed as inches of water gauge (w.g.)

ρ is the air or gas density, expressed as pounds per cubic foot $\left(\frac{lbm}{ft^3}\right)$

Use: To describe the relationship between the velocity pressure (VP), (kinetic pressure) of a ventilation system, the density of the air or gas, and the duct velocity.

Note: The denominator term can either be expressed directly as the density of a gas, or as a multiplier of a standard or given density.

Example:

What is velocity of air flowing through a duct with a velocity pressure of 4.1 inches w.g. and a density of $0.69 \left(\frac{lbm}{ft^3}\right)$?

$$V = 1096 \sqrt{\frac{VP}{\rho}}$$

$$VP = 4.1 \; inches \; \text{w. g.}$$
$$\rho = 0.69 \left(\frac{lbm}{ft^3}\right)$$

Step 1: Solve for V

$$V = 1096 \sqrt{\frac{4.1 \; inches \; \text{w. g.}}{0.69 \left(\frac{lbm}{ft^3}\right)}}$$

$$V = 2{,}671.64 \; fpm$$

Average Duct Velocity Pressure

$$VP_{ave} = \left(\frac{\sqrt{VP_1} + \sqrt{VP_2} + \cdots \sqrt{VP_n}}{n}\right)^2$$

Where:

VP_{ave} is the average velocity pressure of a duct, expressed as inches of water gauge (w.g.)

VP_1 is the velocity pressure measured at point 1 of a traverse, expressed as inches of water gauge (w.g.)

VP_2 is the velocity pressure measured at point 2 of a traverse, expressed as inches of water gauge (w.g.)

VP_n is the velocity pressure measured at point n of a traverse, expressed as inches of water gauge (w.g.)

n is the number of VP measurements during a traverse. At least 6 points for small round ducts (<6" diameter), and as many as 20 points for very large ducts or stacks.

Use: A method to calculate the average duct velocity pressure (VP_{ave}) based on the individual velocity pressures (VP) measured during a pitot traverse.

Example:

A Pitot traverse of a round, 4-inch duct yielded the following velocity pressures:

0.72, 0.72, 0.75, 0.79, 0.82, 0.87

Calculate the average velocity pressure.

$$VP_{ave} = \left(\frac{\sqrt{VP_1} + \sqrt{VP_2} + \cdots \sqrt{VP_n}}{n}\right)^2$$

$$VP_{ave} = \left(\frac{\sqrt{0.72} + \sqrt{0.72} + \sqrt{0.75} + \sqrt{0.79} + \sqrt{0.82} + \sqrt{0.87}}{6}\right)^2$$

$$VP_{ave} = \left(\frac{0.85 + 0.85 + 0.87 + 0.89 + 0.91 + 0.93}{6}\right)^2$$

$$VP_{ave} = 0.78 \; inches \; \text{w.g.}$$

Resultant Duct Velocity Pressure

$$VP_r = \left(\frac{Q_1}{Q_3}\right)VP_1 + \left(\frac{Q_2}{Q_3}\right)VP_2$$

Where:
VP_r is the resultant velocity pressure, expressed as inches of water gauge (w.g.)
VP_1 is the velocity pressure in branch 1, expressed as inches of water gauge (w.g.)
VP_2 is the velocity pressure in branch 2, expressed as inches of water gauge (w.g.)
Q_1 is the volumetric flow rate in branch 1, expressed as (CFM)
Q_2 is the volumetric flow rate in branch 2, expressed as (CFM)
Q_3 is the volumetric flow rate in the main duct, expressed as (CFM)

Use: To correct for velocity changes between branches and the main duct. The resultant velocity pressure (VP_r), corresponds to the 'velocity' of the two volumetric flow rates of the branches.

Example:
To determine if a correction to the system is needed, the resultant velocity pressure must be calculated. There are two duct branches entering a main duct. The volumetric flow rate in branch **1** is 700 CFM, branch **2** is 900 CFM, and the main duct is 1,600 CFM. The velocity pressure in branch **1** is 0.90 inches w.g. and the velocity pressure in branch **2** is 0.75 inches w.g.. Calculate the resultant velocity pressure

$$VP_r = \left(\frac{Q_1}{Q_3}\right)VP_1 + \left(\frac{Q_2}{Q_3}\right)VP_2$$

$$Q_1 = 700 \; CFM \qquad\qquad VP_1 = 0.90 \; inches \; W.G.$$
$$Q_2 = 900 \; CFM \qquad\qquad VP_2 = 0.75 \; inches \; W.G.$$
$$Q_3 = 1,600 \; CFM$$

Step 1: Solve for VP_r

$$VP_r = \left(\frac{Q_1}{Q_3}\right)VP_1 + \left(\frac{Q_2}{Q_3}\right)VP_2$$

$$VP_r = \left(\frac{700 \; CFM}{1,600 \; CFM}\right)0.90 \; inches \; W.G. + \left(\frac{900 \; CFM}{1,600 \; CFM}\right)0.75 \; inches \; W.G.$$

$$VP_r = 0.39 + 0.42$$

$$VP_r = 0.81 \; inches \; w.g.$$

If the velocity pressure in the main duct is less than VP_r, then no correction is necessary.

Balancing Flow Rate at Junctions Using SP

$$Q_{corr} = Q_{lower} \sqrt{\frac{SP_{gov}}{SP_{lower}}}$$

Where:

Q_{corr} is the corrected (adjusted) volumetric flow through the duct of lower resistance, expressed as (CFM)

Q_{lower} is the original (designed or current) volumetric flow through the duct of lower resistance, expressed as (CFM)

SP_{gov} is the static pressure of the duct with the larger loss (governing), expressed as inches of water gauge (w.g.)

SP_{lower} is the static pressure of the duct with the smaller loss, expressed as inches of water gauge (w.g.)

Use: To balance a system at branches using static pressure. Adjust the flow rate so that the static pressure is balanced with the duct that has the highest static pressure during the design process.

Example:

The design shows two ducts meeting at a junction. Duct 1 is designed to flow 500 CFM and has a calculated static pressure of 1.05 inches w.g., and duct 2 is designed to flow 400 CFM and has a calculated static pressure of 0.9 inches w.g.. Is the system balanced? If not, what should be done?

Step 1: Determine the SP ratio

$$\frac{1.05 - 0.9}{1.05} = 14\%$$

Because the difference is greater than 5% adjustments should be made

Calculate the corrected flow rate

$$Q_{corr} = Q_{lower} \sqrt{\frac{SP_{gov}}{SP_{lower}}}$$

$$Q_{lower} = 400\ CFM$$
$$SP_{gov} = 1.05\ inches\ w.\,g.$$
$$SP_{lower} = 0.9\ inches\ w.\,g.$$

$$Q_{corr} = 400\ CFM \sqrt{\frac{1.05\ inches\ w.\,g.}{0.9\ inches\ w.\,g.}}$$

$$Q_{corr} = 432\ CFM$$

Use this value for flow rate for any remaining design calculations for the system.

Conservation of Energy- Including Losses

$$SP_1 + VP_1 = SP_2 + VP_2 + h_L$$

Where:

VP is the velocity pressure, which is the kinetic pressure in the direction of flow, expressed as inches of water gauge (w.g.).

SP is the static pressure, which is the potential pressure exerted in all directions by a fluid at rest, expressed as inches of water gauge (w.g.).

h_L is the energy losses encountered by the air as it flows from upstream to downstream points, expressed as inches of water gauge (w.g.).

Note: The subscript 1 is a point upstream and the subscript 2 is a point downstream

Use: To describe the conservation of energy in an industrial ventilation system by accounting for all energy (friction) losses that occur within a duct or into a hood, as air flows from an upstream to a downstream point. The formula above expresses this concept in terms of pressure.

Also written as:

$$SP_1 + VP_1 = SP_2 + VP_2 + \Sigma_{Losses\ 1-2}$$

Example:

Calculate the energy loss downstream when the velocity pressure is 1.3 inches w.g. and the upstream static pressure is 1.9 inches w.g.?

$$SP_1 + VP_1 = SP_2 + VP_2 + h_L$$

Step 1: Rearrange the equation

If there are no energy losses associated with hood entry, then:

$$SP_1 = SP_2, which\ is\ 1.9\ inches\ w.g.\ and\ VP_1\ and\ VP_1 = VP_2, which\ is\ 1.3\ inches\ w.g.$$

$$SP_2 = -VP_2 - h_L$$

Step 2: Solve for h_L

$$h_L = -SP_2 - VP_2$$

$$h_L = -(-1.9\ inches\ w.g.) - 1.3\ inches\ w.g.$$

$$h_L = 0.6\ inches\ w.g.$$

Hood Entry Coefficient

$$C_e = \sqrt{\frac{VP}{|SP_h|}}$$

Where:

C_e is the hood entry coefficient. It is an alternate method for describing hood entry losses. (unitless)

VP is the velocity pressure, which is the kinetic pressure in the direction of flow, expressed as inches of water gauge (w.g.)

SP_h is the hood static pressure, measured by a U-tube manometer and expressed as inches of water gauge (w.g.)

Use: To determine the relationship between the velocity (kinetic) pressure (VP) and static (potential) pressure (SP) in a ventilation system, and how the ratio provides an indication of the overall efficiency (C_e), of the system.

Note: If there are no losses, then SP_h = VP and C_e = 1.00. However, as hoods always have some losses, C_e is always less than 1.00.

Example:

Calculate the hood entry coefficient for a hood with air flow velocity pressure of 1.2 inches w.g. and a hood static pressure of -1.5 inches w.g.

$$C_e = \sqrt{\frac{VP}{|SP_h|}}$$

$$VP = 1.2\ inches\ W.G.$$
$$SP_h = -1.5\ inches\ W.G.$$

Step 1: Solve for C_e

$$C_e = \sqrt{\frac{1.2\ inches\ w.g.}{|-1.5\ inches\ w.g.|}}$$

$$C_e = 0.89$$

Hood Entry Loss

$$h_e = \frac{1 - C_e^2}{C_e^2} VP$$

Where:

h_e is the hood entry energy loss due to pressure and friction, expressed as inches of water gauge (w.g.)

C_e is the hood entry coefficient. It is an alternate method for describing hood entry losses. (unitless)

VP is the velocity pressure, which is the kinetic pressure in the direction of flow, expressed as inches of water gauge (w.g.)

Use: To calculate the hood entry (energy) loss for air entering a hood.

Example:

Calculate the hood entry loss factor for a hood with air flowing through a plain opening, and resulting in a duct velocity pressure of 0.75 inches w.g.

$$h_e = \frac{1 - C_e^2}{C_e^2} VP$$

$$C_e = 0.72$$

$$VP = 0.75 \; inches \; w.g.$$

Step 1: Solve for h_e

$$h_e = \frac{1 - C_e^2}{C_e^2} VP$$

$$h_e = \frac{1 - (0.72)^2}{(0.72)^2} (.75 \; inches \; w.g.)$$

$$h_e = 0.70 \; inches \; w.g.$$

Hood Static Pressure

$$|SP_h| = VP + h_e$$

Where:

$|SP_h|$ is the absolute value of the hood static pressure, expressed as inches of water gauge (w.g.)

VP is the velocity pressure, which is the kinetic pressure in the direction of flow, expressed as inches of water gauge (w.g.)

h_e is the hood entry energy loss due to pressure and friction, expressed as inches of water gauge (w.g.)

Use: To describe the energy loss that occurs as air is accelerated and enters a hood.

Note: The hood entry loss (h_e) is expressed as a hood loss factor (f_h) multiplied by the duct velocity pressure (VP).

$$h_e = F_h VP$$

F_h values are provided for different hood types in the ACGIH literature. The loss factor may also be designated as K, which can be applied to hood or duct calculations.

Example:

Estimate the hood static pressure if the velocity pressure of 1.0 inch w.g., and according to literature, the hood entry loss factor for a plain round opening is 0.93.

$$|SP_h| = VP + h_e$$

$$h_e = F_h VP$$

Step 1: Solve for $|SP_h|$

$$|SP_h| = 1.0 \ inches \ \mathrm{w.g.} + 0.93$$

$$|SP_h| = 1.93 \ inches \ \mathrm{w.g.}$$

Example:

Estimate the hood entry loss factor if static pressure is determined to be -2.0 inches w.g. and the velocity pressure 1.0 inches w.g.

$$|SP_h| = VP + h_e$$

$$|-2.0| = 1.0 + h_e$$

$$h_e = |-2.0| - 1.0$$

$$= 1.0 \ \mathrm{inches} \ \mathrm{w.g.}$$

Volumetric Flow - Hood Entry Loss Factor (F_h) and Hood Static Pressure (SP_h)

$$Q = 1096A \sqrt{\frac{SP_h}{\rho(1 + F_h)}}$$

Where:

Q is the volumetric flow rate, expressed as actual cubic feet per minute (CFM)

A is the cross-sectional area of the duct, expressed as square feet (ft^2)

ρ is the air or gas density, expressed as pounds per cubic foot $\left(\frac{lbm}{ft^3}\right)$

SP_h is the hood static pressure, expressed as inches of water gauge (w.g.)

F_h is the hood entry loss factor (unitless)

Use: The hood static pressure methods of estimating air flow into an exhaust hood or duct.

For Standard Air, the equation becomes

$$Q = 4005A \sqrt{\frac{SP_h}{df(1 + F_h)}}$$

Note: The density of air is 1.

Where:

Q is the volumetric flow rate, expressed as actual cubic feet per minute (CFM)

A is the cross-sectional area of the duct, expressed as square feet (ft^2)

SP_h is the hood static pressure, expressed as inches of water gauge (w.g.)

F_h is the hood entry loss factor (unitless)

df is the is the density correction factor

Example:
Calculate the volumetric flow rate of air (at standard conditions) through a ten-inch diameter duct if the hood static pressure is 1.2 inches w.g.?

Note: The hood is considered a plain opening with a hood entry loss factor of 0.93.

Step 1: Find the Area of the Duct

$$A = \pi r^2$$

$$A = \pi \left(\frac{5}{12}\right)^2$$

$$A = 0.54 \, ft^2$$

Step 2: Solve for Q

$$Q = 4005A \sqrt{\frac{SP_h}{(1 + F_h)}}$$

$$Q = 4005(0.54 \, ft^2) \sqrt{\frac{1.2 \, inches \, W.G.}{(1 + 0.93)}}$$

$$Q = 2184 \, ft^2 \, x \, 0.788 \, inches \, W.G.$$

$$Q = 1720 \, CFM$$

Effective Ventilation Rate

$$Q' = \frac{Q}{m_i}$$

Where:

Q' is the effective ventilation rate, which is the flow that dilutes the contaminant to acceptable levels, expressed as (CFM)

Q is the actual dilution ventilation rate, expressed as (CFM)

m_i is the safety factor, ranging 1 to 10, also known as mixing factor. If greater than 5, dilution ventilation may not be effective

Use: To control the level of airborne contaminants to some acceptable room concentration by introducing outside air to the space to dilute and maintain an acceptable concentration.

Example:

The engineer designed the air system to provide dilution ventilation of 2500 CFM to control a contaminant concentration to the Permissible Exposure Limit (PEL) under ideal conditions. The industrial hygienist recognizes that that the room is crowded with poor supply locations, and requests a mixing factor of 2. Calculate the effective ventilation rate.

$$Q' = \frac{Q}{m_i}$$

Step 1: Solve for Q'

$$Q' = \frac{2500\ CFM}{2}$$

$$Q' = 1250\ CFM$$

Accordingly, the actual ventilation rate should be increased to account for the mixing conditions (safety factor).

Air Changes per Hour

$$N_{changes} = \frac{60Q}{V_r}$$

Where:

V_r is the volume of the room, expressed as (ft^3)

60 converts minutes to hours for N

$N_{changes}$ is the number of room air changes per hour (ACH)

Use: To calculate the number of room air changer per hour (N), based the volume of a room (V), and the dilution ventilation rate (Q)

Example:

Calculate the number of air changes per hour that occur in a storage chamber that is 30 feet wide, 20 feet long, and 10 feet high. The chamber is provided with 2200 CFM of clean air.

Step 1: Calculate the chamber volume

$$V_r = 30\ feet\ x\ 20\ feet\ x\ 10\ feet$$

$$V_{chamber} = 6,000\ ft^3$$

Step 2: Calculate $N_{changes}$

$$N_{changes} = \frac{60Q}{V_r}$$

$$Q = 2,200\ CFM$$

$$V_r = 6,000\ ft^3$$

$$N_{changes} = \frac{60(2,200\ CFM)}{6,000\ ft^3}$$

$$N_{changes} = 22.0\ ACH$$

Dilution Equation

$$Q = \frac{403(S.G.)(ER)(mi)(10^6)}{(MW)(C_g)}$$

Where:
Q is the volumetric flow rate, expressed as cubic feet per minute (CFM)
S.G. is the specific gravity of a volatile liquid

ER is the evaporation rate of liquid, expressed as pints per minute $\left(\frac{pints}{minute}\right)$

MW is the molecular weight of liquid
C_g is the concentration target, expressed as parts per million (ppm)
m_i is a safety factor, also known as the mixing factor (unitless)

Use: Describes the calculation for the amount of dilution air (Q), needed to maintain a steady state concentration of contaminant.

$$Q = \frac{24(S.G.)(ER)(mi)(10^6)}{(MW)(C_g)}$$

Q is the volumetric flow rate, expressed as (M^3/sec)
ER is the evaporation rate of liquid, expressed as (L/sec)

Example:
Methyl chloroform is lost by evaporation from a tank at a rate of 1.5 pints per 60 minutes. What is the effective ventilation rate (Q) and the actual ventilation rate required to maintain the vapor concentration at the TLV?

$$Q = \frac{403(S.G.)(ER)(mi)(10^6)}{(MW)(C_g)}$$

$$S.G. = 1.32$$

$$ER = \frac{1.5\ pints}{60\ minutes}$$

$$m_i = 5$$

$$MW = 133.4$$

$$TLV = 350\ ppm$$

Step 1: Solve for Q

$$Q = \frac{403(\text{S.G.})(\text{ER})(mi)(10^6)}{(\text{MW})(C_g)}$$

$$Q = \frac{403(1.32)(\frac{1.5\ pints}{60\ minutes})(5)(10^6)}{(133.4)(350ppm)}$$

$$Q = 1,425\ CFM$$

Concentration Over Time (Purging)

$$C = C_o e^{-t\,N\,changes}$$

Where:

C is the final airborne concentration of contaminant, expressed as the decimal equivalent for parts per million

C_O is the initial airborne concentration of the contaminant, expressed as the decimal equivalent for parts per million

t is the amount of time that room has purged, expressed as (hr)

N is the number of air changes for the room per hour (ACH)

e is the natural logarithm (2.718)

V shown below is the room volume, expressed as (ft^3)

Use: Describes the relationship between the decrease in the concentration of a contaminant in a room over time (purging) when the active generation of the contaminant has concluded.

Note: The equation below calculates the number of room air changes per hour

$$N = \frac{Q'60}{V} = \frac{\frac{ft^3}{min} x \frac{60\,min}{hr}}{ft^3} = ACH$$

Example:

Calculate the final room concentration of toluene after 15 minutes, if the initial concentration was 100 ppm. The contaminant release is complete and fully evaporated. The measure dilution ventilation creates of 25 air changes per hour. The room is 20 feet, by 40 feet, by 12 feet.

$$C = C_o e^{-t\,N\,changes}$$

$$C_o = 100\ ppm$$

$$t = \left(\frac{15\ min}{\frac{60\ min}{hr}} \right) = 0.25\ \text{hours}$$

$$N = \frac{25\ changes}{hr}$$

Step 1: Calculate the e and exponent value

$$e^{-.25x25}$$
$$= e^{-6.3}$$
$$= 0.0019$$

Step 2: Solve for C

$$C = C_o e^{-t\,N\,changes}$$

$$C = 100e^{-6.3}$$

$$C = 0.2\ ppm$$

Concentration Buildup when the Initial Concentration is Zero

$$C = \frac{G}{Q'}\left(1 - e^{\frac{-Nt}{60}}\right) x\ 10^6$$

Where:

C is the concentration of the contaminant gas or vapor, expressed as (ppm)

G is the generation rate of the contaminant gas or vapor, expressed as (CFM)

Q' is the effective volumetric flow rate of clean dilution air, expressed as(CFM)

N is the number of air changes in the room per hour, expressed as (ACH)

60 is the minutes to hours conversion factor

V shown below is the room volume, expressed as (ft^3)

t is the specified amount of time, expressed as minutes

Use: Describes the relationship between the generation rate (G) of an airborne vapor or gas and the contaminant buildup (C) after a specified time interval (t) when the initial concentration is zero.

Note: The equations below calculate the number of room air changes per hour.

$$N_{changes} = \frac{60Q}{V_r} \quad \text{or previously, } N = \frac{Q'60}{V} = \frac{\frac{ft^3}{min} x \frac{60\ min}{hr}}{ft^3} = ACH$$

Example:

In a room with no initial airborne levels, what will the room concentration of isobutyl alcohol be after 15 minutes if the vapor is generated at a rate of 3 CFM in a room measuring 15 feet x 45 x 12 feet while being ventilated with clean dilution air at a flow of 2,200 CFM?

Step 1: Calculate Room Volume

$$15\ feet\ x\ 45\ feet\ x\ 12\ feet = 8,100\ ft^3$$

Step 2: Calculate N

$$Q' = 2,200\ CFM$$
$$V = 8,100\ ft^3$$

$$N = \frac{Q'60}{V} = \frac{\frac{ft^3}{min} x \frac{60\ min}{hr}}{ft^3} = ACH$$

$$N = \frac{Q'60}{V} = \frac{\frac{2,200\ ft^3}{min} x \frac{60\ min}{hr}}{8,100\ ft^3}$$

$$N = \frac{132{,}000\ \frac{ft^3}{hr}}{8{,}100\ ft^3}$$

$$N = 16.3\ ACH$$

Step 3: Calculate C

$$G = 3\ CFM$$
$$Q' = 2{,}200\ CFM$$
$$N = -16.3\ ACH$$
$$t = 15\ minutes$$

$$C = \frac{G}{Q'}\left(1 - e^{\frac{-Nt}{60}}\right)x\ 10^6$$

$$C = \frac{3\ CFM}{2{,}200\ CFM}\left[1 - e^{-16.3\frac{changes}{hour}}(15\ minutes)/60\frac{minutes}{hour}\right]x\ 10^6$$

$$C = 0.0013(1 - e^{-4.1})\ x\ 10^6$$

$$C = (0.0013)(1 - 0.017)\ x\ 10^6$$

$$C = (0.0013)(0.983)\ x\ 10^6$$

$$C = 1{,}277\ ppm$$

Time Interval of Purging

$$t_2 - t_1 = -\frac{V_r}{Q'} \ln\left(\frac{C_{g2}}{C_{g1}}\right)$$

Where:

t_2 - t_1 is the change in time (Δt), the time interval, expressed as minutes
V_r is the room volume, expressed as (ft^3)
Q' is the effective dilution ventilation rate, expressed as (CFM)
ln is the natural logarithm
C_{g1} is the initial airborne concentration of the contaminant
C_{g2} is the final airborne concentration of the contaminant, expressed as (ppm)

Use: To determine the time interval needed to decrease (purge) the room concentration of a contaminant when the active generation of contaminant has stopped, and the room is still being ventilated with clean dilution air.

Example:
The initial concentration of toluene is 100 ppm in a room that is 20 feet by 35 by 15 feet and supplied with 2,200 CFM of clean dilution air. Calculate the time needed to reduce the concentration to 10 ppm if the toluene is no longer being released?

Step 1: Calculate V_r

$$20 \, feet \; x \; 35 \, feet \; x \; 15 \, feet = 10{,}500 \, ft^3$$

Step 2: Calculate Δt

$$t_2 - t_1 = -\frac{V_r}{Q'} \ln\left(\frac{C_2}{C_1}\right)$$

$$V_r = 10{,}500 \, ft^3$$
$$Q' = 2{,}200 \, CFM$$
$$C_2 = 10 \, ppm$$
$$C_1 = 100 \, ppm_1$$

$$t_2 - t_1 = -\frac{10{,}500 \, ft^3}{2{,}200 \, CFM} \ln\left(\frac{10 \, ppm}{100 \, ppm_1}\right)$$

$$\Delta t = -4.77x \, ln \; 0.1$$

$$\Delta t = 11.0 \, minutes$$

Contaminant Concentration Buildup

$$ln\frac{(G - Q'C_2)}{(G - Q'C_1)} = -\frac{Q'(t_2 - t_1)}{V_r}$$

Where:

G is the generation rate (leak or evaporation) of a gas or vapor, expressed as (CFM)

Q' is the effective flow rate of clean dilution air supplied to the room (CFM)

V_r is the room volume (ft^3)

C_1 is the initial airborne contaminant concentration (decimal equivalent of ppm)

C_2 is the final airborne contaminant concentration (decimal equivalent of ppm)

t_1 is the initial time related to C_1 (minutes)

t_2 is the final time of the occurrence of C_2 (minutes)

ln is the natural logarithm

Use: To determine the relationship between the contaminant concentration buildup actively being generated at any point in time.

Example:

Calculate the final room concentration of butyl alcohol after 12 minutes if the vapor is generated at a rate of 7 CFM in a room that is 15 feet by 50 feet long by 10 feet. The initial measured concentration was 50 ppm. The volumetric flow of clean dilution air is 2,200 CFM.

$$ln\frac{(G - Q'C_2)}{(G - Q'C_1)} = -\frac{Q'(t_2 - t_1)}{V_{room}}$$

$G = 7\ CFM$

$Q' = 2,500\ CFM$

$t_2 - t_1 = 12\ minutes$

Step 1: Calculate C_1

$$C_1 = 50\ ppm\ x\ 10^{-6} = 0.00005\ \text{(the decimal equivalent)}$$

Step 2: Calculate the room volume:

$$V = 15\ feet\ x\ 50\ feet\ x\ 10\ feet = 7{,}500 ft^3$$

Step 3: Solve for C_2

$$ln\frac{(G - Q'C_2)}{(G - Q'C_1)} = -\frac{Q'(t_2 - t_1)}{V_{room}}$$

$$ln\frac{(7\ CFM - 2{,}200\ CFM(C_2))}{(7\ CFM - 2{,}200\ CFM(0.00005))} = -\frac{2{,}200\ CFM(12\ minutes)}{7{,}500\ ft^3}$$

$$ln\frac{(7\ CFM - 2{,}200\ CFM\ (C_2))}{6.89\ CFM} = -3.52$$

Note: To mathematically remove the natural log (ln), take the antilog (e^x) of both sides.

$$\frac{(7\ CFM - 2{,}200\ CFM\ (C_2))}{6.89\ CFM} = 0.03$$

$$7\ CFM - 2{,}200\ CFM(C_2) = 0.207$$

$$-2{,}200\ CFM\ (C_2) = -6.79$$

$$C_2 = 0.003$$

$$0.0031\ x10^6\ \text{(to change from decimal equivalent to ppm)}$$

$$C_2 = 3{,}000\ ppm$$

Rubric 7: Engineering Control and Ventilation Questions

1. Industrial processes and ventilation systems often need more air than is called for in the original design documents; V-belt drives are commonly used on fans for these applications. Improperly aligned and tensioned V-belt drives can reduce air flow by what percentage of design air flow?

    A) 30% to 40%.
    B) 50% to 60%.
    C) 10% to 20%.
    D) No reduction.

2. A researcher in a laboratory wants to add a fume hood to the laboratory. The hood has a 6-foot-wide sash and can be safely operated at sash height of 18 inches. The laboratory site safety manual stipulates that 80 FPM is the minimum allowable fume hood face velocity. Assuming a 10% safety factor, what is the minimum additional volume of make-up air to be supplied to the laboratory in order for the fume hood to function safely?

    A) 9 CFM.
    B) 80 CFM.
    C) 720 CFM.
    D) 792 CFM.

3. An exhaust fan was selected for a particular industrial process to exhaust 40,000 CFM against a system static pressure of 4.0 inches w.g. when operating at 1,600 RPM and developing 20 BHP. Upon installation, it was discovered that the fan was actually exhausting 50,000 CFM. Use the fan law(s) to calculate the new BHP developed. RPM 2 = 1,280 RPM

    A) 10.2 BHP.
    B) 12.4 BHP.
    C) 16.6 BHP.
    D) 18.8 BHP.

4. A fan selected to operate at 9000 CFM, 1,500 RPM, requiring 5 BHP at 1 inch w.g. After installation, the process required an additional 2,000 CFM of air to make production target. Using the fan law(s), calculate the new speed, pressure and brake horsepower requirements.

    A) 1560 RPM, 1.5 inches WG, 6.5 BHP.
    B) 1650 RPM, 1.6 inches WG, 7.7 BHP.
    C) 1833 RPM, 1.5 inches WG, 9.1 BHP.
    D) 1833 RPM, 3.2 inches WG, 10.8 BHP.

5. The IH has asked the maintenance department for the air flow through a 12-inch diameter round duct. The senior maintenance person performs a 6-point pitot traverse and obtains the following values: 1.5, 1.4, 1.4, 1.3, 1.3, 1.2. The maintenance person provides this information to the IH and goes home. Calculate the air flow through the duct.

   A) 3618 CFM.
   B) 4639 FPM.
   C) 4005 CFM.
   D) 3700 FPM.

6. What is the friction loss in 20 feet of 10-inch diameter round galvanized duct based on a velocity of 2000 FPM and nomograph values of $K = 2.4$ per 100 ft. and a VP of 0.25 in WG?

   A) 2 friction loss units.
   B) 50 inches WG.
   C) 1.9 inches WG.
   D) 0.12 inches WG.

7. The laboratory hood operation plan requires the average face velocity to be between 90 and 110 FPM. With the sash open on the hood (18 inches) and with no by-pass feature, the average face velocity is 190 FPM. What height should the sash be set to in order to have a face velocity of 100 FPM?

   A) 8 inches.
   B) 31.1 inches.
   C) 34.2 inches.
   D) 36 inches.

8. A manometer on the suction side of a fan is reading 0.59 inches WG velocity pressure and -1.3 inches WG static pressure. What is the total pressure on the suction side of the fan?

   A) 0.47 inches WG.
   B) 0.71 inches WG.
   C) -0.47 inches WG.
   D) -0.71 inches WG.

9. What is the hood entry coefficient for a hood with air flow velocity pressure of 1.5 inches WG and a hood static pressure of 1.8 inches WG?

   A) 0.20.
   B) 0.57.
   C) 0.91.
   D) 1.47.

10. While performing a ventilation evaluation in an old facility, an IH must determine the flow through a large duct. A tape measure is looped around the duct yielding a result of 70 inches. The average velocity pressure is 1.2 inches WG. Calculate the flow.

    A) 11,845 CFM.
    B) 11,845 FPM.
    C) 4387 CFM.
    D) 4387 FPM.

11. The ventilation system was designed for a duct velocity of at least 5000 FPM to transport particulates to the storage hopper. The air flow is specified at 3200 CFM. Calculate the best duct size to meet the needs of the system.

    A) 10 inch.
    B) 11 inch.
    C) 14 inch.
    D) 18 inch.

12. An exhaust system is operating on a process with the exhaust stream temperature of 150° F. A literature search reveals that the air density correction factor at this temperature and 1 atmosphere of pressure is 0.87. The velocity pressure has been measured at 2.5 inches WG. Calculate the air velocity in the system.

    A) 6124 FPM.
    B) 6328 FPM.
    C) 6784 FPM.
    D) 6880 FPM.

13. A Class 1 biosafety cabinet has two arm openings that are open (not equipped with gloves). The arm openings are round and have a diameter of 8 inches. The cabinet specifies a minimum face velocity of 75 FPM. Calculate the airflow required to meet the face velocity requirement.

    A) 26 CFM.
    B) 53 CFM.
    C) 51 CFM.
    D) 75 CFM.

14. Which of the following is NOT considered one of the five components of a local exhaust system?

    A) Hood.
    B) Magnehelic gauge.
    C) Air cleaner.
    D) Ductwork.

15. Select the best description of losses as related to a local exhaust ventilation system.

    A) Hood entry, friction, potential energy.
    B) Friction, elbow, potential energy.
    C) Elbow, friction, air cleaner.
    D) Kinetic, frenetic, potential energy.

16. Brake horse power is the AHP divided by the mechanical efficiency. Calculate the BHP for this system: FTP = 2.0 inches WG, Q = 1200 CFM, ME = 0.5. Assume STP.

    A) 1
    B) 600
    C) 300
    D) 0.76

17. Select the answer that best describes the ASHRAE 55 80-20-10 recommendation.

    A) 80% of the air can be recirculated if 20% of the air is from an outside source, and contaminants are less than 10% of any occupational exposure limit.
    B) If 80% of the occupants are satisfied with all environmental conditions, or if less than 20% are dissatisfied, then comfort conditions have been met. If more than 10% are dissatisfied with any one condition, such as temperature, odors, humidity or drafts, then satisfactory comfort conditions have not been achieved.
    C) Relative humidity must be maintained between 20% and 80% with 10% of the air from an outside source.
    D) Office environments should not exceed 80% of occupancy load more than 20% of the day, and the optimum conditions are equal to or less than 10% of the day.

18. Calculate the energy loss at a certain downstream point if the velocity pressure is 1.4 inches WG and the upstream static pressure is 1.8 inches WG.

    A) -1.45 inches WG.
    B) -0.96 inches WG.
    C) 0.4 inches WG.
    D) 1.23 inches WG.

19. What is the final room concentration of acetone if the vapor is generated at a rate of 8 CFM while the room is being ventilated with dilution air containing 40 PPM of acetone at a flow of 2,700 CFM?

    A) 3,003 PPM.
    B) 4,653 PPM.
    C) 5,908 PPM.
    D) 8,851 PPM.

20. What type of air velocity instrument is utilized to gather data on static pressures and linear velocities?

    A) Rotating Vane Anemometer.
    B) Thermal Anemometer.
    C) Swinging Vane Anemometer.
    D) U-Tube Manometer.

Rubric 7: Engineering Control and Ventilation Answers

1. Answer C.
   Explanation: Improperly aligned and tensioned V-belt drives can reduce air flow by 10% to 20% of design air flow. *Source: The New York Blower Company Engineering Letters, Letter 6, 1996*

2. Answer D.
   Explanation:
   Known
   V = 80 FPM
   A = (6ft. X 1.5ft) = 9 ft^2

$$Q = VA$$

$$Q = 1.1 \, x \, (80 \, fpm \, x \, 9 \, ft^2)$$

$$Q = 792 \, CFM$$

3. Answer A.
   Explanation:

$$\frac{BHP \, 1}{BHP \, 2} = \left(\frac{RPM \, 1}{RPM2}\right)^3$$

$$\frac{20}{BHP \, 2} = \left(\frac{1,600}{1,280}\right)^3$$

$$BHP \, 2 = \frac{20}{\left(\frac{1,600}{1,280}\right)^3}$$

$$BHP \, 2 = 10.2 \, BHP$$

4. Answer C.
   Explanation:

$$CFM\ 2 = 9{,}000\ CFM + 2{,}000\ CFM = 11{,}000\ CFM$$

$$\frac{RPM\ 2}{RPM\ 1} = \frac{CFM\ 2}{CFM\ 1}$$

$$RPM\ 2 = RPM\ 1\left(\frac{CFM\ 2}{CFM\ 1}\right) = 1{,}500\ x\ \frac{11{,}000\ CFM}{9{,}000\ CFM}$$

$$RPM\ 2 = 1{,}833\ RPM$$

$$\frac{P\ 2}{P\ 1} = \left(\frac{RPM\ 2}{RPM\ 1}\right)^2$$

$$P\ 2 = P1\left(\frac{RPM\ 2}{RPM\ 1}\right)^2$$

$$P\ 2 = 1.0\left(\frac{1{,}833\ RPM}{1{,}500\ RPM}\right)^2$$

$$P\ 2 = 1.5\ inches\ wg$$

$$\frac{BHP\ 2}{BHP\ 1} = \left(\frac{RPM\ 2}{RPM\ 1}\right)^3$$

$$BHP\ 2 = BHP\ 1\left(\frac{RPM\ 2}{RPM\ 1}\right)^3$$

$$BHP\ 2 = 5\ BHP\left(\frac{1{,}833\ RPM}{1{,}500\ RPM}\right)^3$$

$$BHP\ 2 = 9.1\ BHP$$

5. Answer A.
   Explanation:
   Step 1: Calculate the average velocity pressure

$$VP_{avg} = \left(\frac{\sqrt{VP_1} + \sqrt{VP_2} + \cdots \sqrt{VP_n}}{n}\right)^2$$

$$VP_{avg} = \left(\frac{\sqrt{1.5} + \sqrt{1.4} + \sqrt{1.4} + \sqrt{1.3} + \sqrt{1.3} + \sqrt{1.2}}{6}\right)^2$$

$$VP_{avg} = \left(\frac{6.95}{6}\right)^2 = 1.34 \text{ inches WG}$$

Step 2: Calculate the velocity

$$V = 4005\sqrt{VP}$$

$$V = 4005\sqrt{1.34}$$

$$V = 4639 \text{ FPM}$$

Step 3: Calculate the area of the 12-inch duct in square feet

$$A = \pi r^2$$

$$A = \pi\left(\frac{6}{12}\right)^2 = 0.78 \text{ ft}^2$$

Step 4: Calculate the volume of air flow, Q

$$Q = VA$$

$$Q = 4639 \; FPM \; x \; 0.78 \; ft^2 = 3618 \text{ CFM}$$

Source: Industrial Occupational Hygiene Calculations: A Professional Reference

6. Answer D.
   Explanation:
   Step 1: Calculate the loss

$$SP_{loss} = \frac{K}{100 \; ft} \, xVPx \; length \; ft$$

$$SP_{loss} = \frac{2.4}{100 \; ft} \, x \; 0.25 \; x \; 20 \; ft = 0.12 \text{ inches WG}$$

Source: Laboratory Ventilation Workbook, Burton

      Copyright©2019 SPAN International Training, LLC

7. Answer C.
    Explanation: It assumed that the air flow remains constant. The width of the hood is also constant. Set up an equality and solve for the height.

$$18 \; inches \; x \; 190 \; FPM = Height_2 \, x \; 100 \; FPM$$

$$\frac{18 \; inches \; x \; 190 \; FPM}{100 \; FPM} = Height_2$$

$Height_2$ = 34.2 inches or 2.85 feet

8. Answer D.
    Explanation:

$$TP = VP + SP$$

VP = 0.59 inches WG
SP = -1.3 inches WG

Step 1: Solve for TP

$$TP = VP + SP$$

$$TP = 0.59 \; inches \; WG \; + (-1.3 \; inches \; WG)$$

$$TP = \; -0.71 \; inches \; WG$$

9. Answer C.
    Explanation:

$$C_e = \sqrt{\frac{VP}{|SP_h|}}$$

$$VP = 1.5 \; inches \; WG$$
$$SP_h = 1.8 \; inches \; WG$$

Step 1: Solve for C_e

$$C_e = \sqrt{\frac{1.5 \; inches \; WG}{1.8 \; inches \; WG}}$$

$$C_e = 0.91$$

10. Answer A.
   Explanation:

Step 1: Calculate the duct radius

$$C = 2\pi r$$

$$70 \text{ inches} = 2\pi r$$

$$\frac{70 \text{ inches}}{6.2283} = r$$

$$11.14 \text{ inches} = r$$

Step 2: Calculate the duct area

$$A = \pi r^2$$

$$A = \pi \left(\frac{11.14 \text{ inches}}{12 \frac{inches}{foot}} \right)^2$$

$$A = 2.7 \text{ ft}^2$$

Step 3: Calculate the velocity

$$V = 4005\sqrt{VP}$$

$$V = 4005\sqrt{1.2}$$

$$V = 4387 \text{ FPM}$$

Step 4: Calculate the flow

$$Q = VA$$

$$Q = 4387 \text{ } FPM \text{ } x 2.7 \text{ } ft^2$$

$$Q = 11,845 \text{ CFM}$$

11. Answer A.
   Explanation:

Step 1: Calculate the area of the duct

$$Q = VA$$

$$3200\ CFM = 5000 FPM(A)$$

$$0.64\ \text{ft}^2 = A$$

Step 2: Calculate the duct diameter

$$A = \pi r^2 \text{ and } 2 \times r = d$$

$$0.64\ \text{ft}^2 = \pi r^2$$

$$\sqrt{\frac{0.64\ ft^2}{\pi}} = r$$

0.45 ft = 5.42 inches = r, and 2 x 5.42 inches = 10.8 inches which is the diameter

To maintain the velocity conditions, select the size duct that does NOT exceed the calculated diameter. In this case, a 10-inch duct diameter.

12. Answer C.
   Explanation:
   Step 1: Calculate the velocity using velocity pressure and density correction

$$V = 1096 \sqrt{\frac{VP}{\rho}}$$

$$V = 1096 \sqrt{\frac{2.5}{0.075 \frac{lbm}{ft^3} \ x\ 0.87}}$$

$$V = 6784 \text{ FPM}$$

13. Answer B.
    Explanation:
    Step 1: Solve for Area

$$A = \pi r^2$$

$$A = \pi \left(\frac{4\ inches}{12\frac{inches}{foot}} \right)^2 = 0.35\ \text{ft}^2$$

Since there are 2 openings, the area equals: 0.7 ft^2

Step 2: Solve for Q

$$Q = VA$$

$$Q = 75\ FPM\ x\ 0.7\ ft^2$$

$$Q = 52.5\ \text{CFM}$$

Source: Laboratory Ventilation Workbook, Burton

14. Answer B.
    Explanation: In addition to the 3 listed, *fan and stack* comprise the 5 components of an LEV system. *Source: IH Workbook, 6th edition, Burton*

15. Answer C.
    Explanation:
    As air moves through a duct, losses are created. Static pressure is converted to heat, vibration, noise, etc. The loss is usually related to velocity pressure as:

$$SP_{loss} = K\ x\ VP\ x\ df$$

Note: Typically expressed as inches WG.
Losses include hood entry, friction, elbow, branch entry, system effects, air cleaner and others.
Source: IH Workbook, 6th edition, Burton

16. Answer D.
    Explanation:

Step 1: Solve for air horse power

$$AHP = \frac{Q\ x\ FTP\ x\ d}{6356}$$

$$AHP = \frac{1200\ x\ 2\ x\ 1}{6356}$$

$$APH = 0.38$$

Step 2: Solve for brake horse power

$$BHP = \frac{AHP}{ME}$$

$$BHP = \frac{0.38}{0.5}$$

$$BHP = 0.76 \text{ hp}$$

Source: IH Workbook, 6th edition, Burton

17. Answer B.

Explanation: Per ASHRAE, if 80% of the occupants are satisfied with all environmental conditions, or if less than 20% are dissatisfied, then comfort conditions have been met. If more than 10% are dissatisfied with any one condition, such as temperature, odors, humidity or drafts, then satisfactory comfort conditions have not been achieved. *Source: IH Workbook, 6th edition, Burton*

18. Answer C.

Explanation: h_L is the energy losses encountered by the air as it flows from upstream to downstream points

$$SP_1 + VP_1 = SP_2 + VP_2 + h_L$$

$$SP_2 = 1.8 \; inches \; WG$$
$$VP_2 = 1.4 \; inches \; WG$$

Step 1: Rearrange the equation

$$\text{Since, } SP_1 = SP_2 \text{ and } VP_1 \text{ and } VP_1 = VP_2, \text{ then}$$

$$SP_2 = -VP_2 - h_L$$

Step 2: Solve for h_L

$$h_L = -SP_2 - VP_2$$

$$h_L = -(-1.8 \; inches \; WG) - 1.4 \; inches \; \text{w. g.}$$

$$h_L = 0.4 \; inches \; WG$$

Source: Industrial-Occupational Hygiene Calculations: A Professional Reference

19. Answer: A

$$C = \left(\frac{G}{Q'} \times 10^6\right) + C_{supply}$$

$$G = 8\,CFM$$
$$Q' = 2,700\,CFM$$
$$C_{supply} = 40\,PPM$$

$$C = \left(\frac{8\,CFM}{2,700\,CFM} \times 10^6\right) + 40\,PPM\,m_{supply}$$

$$C = 3,003\,PPM$$

Source: Industrial-Occupational Hygiene Calculations: A Professional Reference

20. Answer C.

Explanation: A swinging vane anemometer is used to check pressures and a wide range of linear velocities. The air velocity instrument is used extensively in field measurements because of its portability, wide scale range, and instantaneous reading features.

Table: Characteristics of Flow Instruments

Instrument	Range (FPM)	Temperature Range
Pitot Tubes with Inclined Manometer	600 and above	0-800 °F
Swinging Vane Anemometers	25-10,000	20-300 °F
Rotating Vane Anemometers	30-10,000	20-150 °F

Source: Industrial Ventilation- A Manual of Recommended Practice, 22nd Edition

Rubric 8: Ergonomics

Ergonomics is the science of fitting work conditions to the capabilities of the worker. The AIHA Ergonomics Committee defines ergonomics as the following:

"A multidisciplinary science that applies principles based on the physical and psychological capabilities of people to the design or modification of jobs, equipment, products, and workplaces. The goals of ergonomics are to decrease risk of injuries and illnesses (especially those related to the musculoskeletal system), to improve worker performance, to decrease worker discomfort, and to improve the quality of work life."

Important Terms and Concepts

Anthropometry – Best described as measuring humans. Typically, straight-line and point to point measurement that includes height, breadth, depth, and distance measurements between landmarks on the body and/or reference surfaces. Designs for consumers historically range between the 5th percentile woman and 95th percentile man.

Biomechanics- The characteristics of the human body described in mechanical terms.

Cumulative trauma disorder (CTD) - A term for syndromes that may or may not show physical manifestations. Characterized by discomfort, pain, or impairment in joints, muscles, tendons, and other soft tissues. Work factors that may cause CTDs include repetition, force and static tension.

Fatigue – The decreased muscular ability to continue an existing effort.

Fitts' Law – Expression of the relation of time and motion expressed in a Motion Time (MT) equation: $MT = a + b \log_2 (2D / W)$.

Lifting Index (LI) – Developed by NIOSH to aid in application of the Recommended Weight Limit (RWL). The equation for calculating the LI: LI = L/RWL, with L the actual load.

Physical Work Capacity – The maximum amount of oxygen that a person can consume in one minute. It is also known as aerobic capacity, maximum aerobic power, and VO_2max.

Recommended Weight Limit (RWL) – Developed by NIOSH. It represents the maximum weight of a load that may be lifted or lowered by about 90 percent of American industrial workers, male or female, who are physically fit and accustomed to physical labor. The equation for calculating the RWL: RWL = LC x HM x VM x DM x AM x FM x CM.

Torque - The product of force and its lever arm to the body joint with the direction of the force perpendicular to its lever arm.

Table: Work Classification Based On Energy Expenditure and Heart Rate

Classification	Total Energy Expenditure (kcal/min)	Heart Rate (beats/min)
Extremely Heavy	15	≥ 160
Very Heavy	10	140
Heavy	7.5	120
Medium	5	100
Light	2.5	≤ 90

Familiarity with the causes, symptoms and physiology of common cumulative trauma disorders (CTDs) is important. The following table describes some of these conditions.

Carpal Tunnel Syndrome - Compression of the median nerve in the carpal tunnel of the wrist.

Cubital Tunnel Syndrome - Compression of the ulnar nerve below the elbow notch.

DeQuervain's Syndrome - Tenosynovitis of the sheath around the abductor and extensor tendons at the base of the thumb.

Epicondylitis (tennis elbow) - Inflammation of tendons that attach to the lateral epicondyle.

Neck Tension Syndrome – Irritation and contraction of the levator scapulae and trapezius muscles of the neck.

Thoracic Outlet Syndrome – Compression between the clavicle and the first and second ribs involving nerves and blood vessels that results in numbness and weakness of the arm.

Trigger Finger - Tenosynovitis that leads to near locking of the tendon.

Raynaud's (white finger) Syndrome – Vascular spasms that result in a lack of blood in the fingers, resulting in cold, numb, white (pale) fingers.

NIOSH Lifting Equation

$$RWL = LC \times HM \times VM \times DM \times AM \times FM \times CM$$

$$RWL\,(lbs) = 51\left(\frac{10}{H}\right)(1 - .0075\,|V - 30|)\left(.82 + \frac{1.8}{D}\right)(1 - (0.0032 \times A))(FM)(CM)$$

$$RWL\,(kg) = 23\left(\frac{25}{H}\right)(1 - .003\,|V - 75|)\left(.82 + \frac{45}{D}\right)(1 - (0.0032 \times A))(FM)(CM)$$

Given

H = Horizontal distance of hands from midpoint between the ankles.
V = Vertical distance of the hand from the floor.
D = Vertical travel distance between origin and destination.
A = Angle of asymmetry, the angular displacement of the load from the sagittal plane in degrees.
F = Average frequency of lift in lifts per minute.

Notes and Modifications:
H = Must be between 10 and 25 inches.
V = Must be between 0 and 70 inches.
V = Is an absolute value indicating the absolute deviation from 30 inches ie; if V = 36 the absolute value would be 6, likewise if V = 24 the absolute value would also be 6.
D = Must be between 10 inches and (70 - V) inches *if less than 10 inches, D = 10.*
F = Must be between .2 (one lift every five minutes) and 15 lifts per minute - duration ranges up to 8 hours.
A = Must be between 0" and 135" angular displacement.

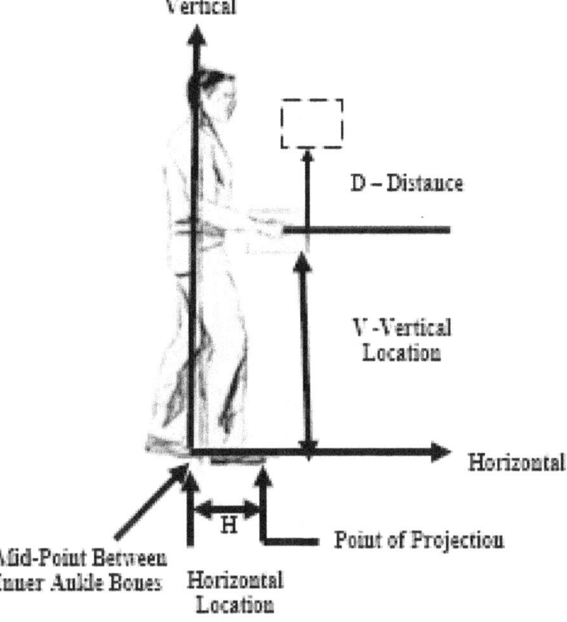

Span image

Rubric 8: Ergonomics Questions

1. The term ergonomics can best be defined as:

   A) Designing equipment and tools for workers.
   B) Developing solutions to reduce work related injuries.
   C) The science of fitting workplace conditions to the capabilities of the working population.
   D) The anticipation, recognition and control of workplace physical hazards.

2. NIOSH draws a distinction between ergonomics and work-related musculoskeletal disorders (WMSDs). Select the best description of WMSDs.

   A) Injuries that involve the physiological and psychological stressors.
   B) Injuries that include the nerves, tendons and supporting structures.
   C) Disorders that effect the general well-being.
   D) Hand-arm vibration syndrome.

3. Which of the following is not a disorder of the upper extremities?

   A) Epicondylitis.
   B) Carpal tunnel syndrome.
   C) Chondromalacia.
   D) Adhesive capsulitis.

4. A condition known as writer's cramp results from compression of the median nerve in the wrist. This condition is also known as:

   A) Cubital Tunnel Syndrome.
   B) Pronator Syndrome.
   C) Raynaud's Syndrome.
   D) Carpal Tunnel Syndrome.

5. Tenosynovitis occurring in the abductor and extensor tendons of the thumb that results in pain and swelling near the base of the thumb is typically diagnosed as:

   A) DeQuervain's Syndrome.
   B) Epicondylitis.
   C) Pronator Syndrome.
   D) Raynaud's Phenomenon.

6. A type of tenosynovitis in which the tendon becomes locked or nearly locked, so that forced movement is jerky, is known as:

   A) Neck Tension Syndrome.
   B) Spasmodic tendonitis.
   C) Thoracic Outlet Syndrome.
   D) Trigger finger.

7. The condition that results from insufficient blood supply, causing blanching and numbness in fingers is known as:

    A) Raynaud's Syndrome.
    B) Trigger finger.
    C) Boney Lacunae Syndrome.
    D) Femoral displacement.

8. Which of the following is not a work-related risk factor for musculoskeletal disorders?

    A) Repetition.
    B) Distribution.
    C) Force.
    D) Posture.

9. Which of the following is not a work-related risk factor for musculoskeletal disorders?

    A) Mechanical stress.
    B) Posture.
    C) Low temperatures.
    D) Resonance.

10. Which of the following is not a work-related risk factor for musculoskeletal disorders?

    A) Static Load.
    B) Mechanical stress.
    C) Vibration.
    D) Anatomy.

11. Which of the following is not a work-related risk factor for musculoskeletal disorders of the lower back?

    A) Anatomy.
    B) Asymmetrical handling.
    C) Repetition.
    D) Handles/coupling.

12. Physiological techniques are useful for repetitive whole-body work. Two human body responses that indicate the extent of the hazard and respond to risk factors are oxygen consumption and heart rate. The oxygen consumed by a person is influenced by the intensity of the task. The rate of oxygen consumption is compared to:

    A) Plyometric capacity.
    B) The Anderson Scale.
    C) The lifting index.
    D) The physical work capacity.

13. In lifting a load, it is important to:

    A) Securely grip the load.
    B) Keep the load close to the body.
    C) Lift slowly and evenly.
    D) All of the above.

14. Carpal tunnel syndrome is:

    A) A respiratory disease resulting from breathing polluted air in tunnels where carbon monoxide is present.
    B) A problem in the wrist resulting from compression of the median nerve.
    C) A common illness of coal miners in the Carpathian Mountains.
    D) An elongation of the finger extensor tendons.

15. Which of the factors noted below is generally not considered to be of significant importance in the causation of cumulative trauma disorders?

    A) Awkward posture.
    B) High hand and finger forces.
    C) Standing work postures.
    D) High frequency or repetition.

16. The application of ergonomics emphasizes:

    A) Selecting and training individuals to fit different jobs.
    B) Designing jobs and tasks to fit people.
    C) Decreasing worker complaint.
    D) Meeting OSHA standards.

17. Back belts:

    A) Are recommended by NIOSH.
    B) Are required by OSHA if back strain is possible.
    C) Have not been shown to lessen the risk of back injury among uninjured workers.
    D) Must be provided at no cost to employees who request them according to OSHA regulations.

18. What is the Recommended Weight Limit (RWL) for the following conditions?

Weight to be lifted = 20 lbs
* Distance between body and hand grip on the object to be lifted = 24 inches
* Vertical position at the beginning of the lift = 36 inches
* Vertical position at end of lift = 46 inches
* Frequency of lift = once every 5 minutes for eight hours

Note: Hand coupling is poor and this job requires a twist from the "eyes front" position of 15°.

A) 14.8 lbs.
B) 16.8 lbs.
C) 20 lbs.
D) 26.8 lbs.

19. Determine the Lifting Index for the following conditions. The recommended weight limit is 14.8 pounds and the load to be lifted is 20 pounds.

A) 0.55
B) 1.35
C) 0.82
D) 0.90

20. Calculate the RWL given the following conditions:

Weight to be lifted = 30 lbs. (13.6 kg)
* Distance between body and hand grip on the object to be lifted = 18 inches (45 cm) Vertical position at the beginning of the lift = 30 inches (75 cm)
* Vertical position at end of lift = 40 inches (100 cm)
* Frequency of lift = once every 5 minutes for one hour

Note: Hand coupling is good, and this activity does not require any twisting movement.

A) 14.0 kg.
B) 12.1 kg.
C) 13.6 kg.
D) 12.8 kg.

Rubric 8: Ergonomics Answers

1. Answer C.
    Explanation: The science of fitting the task or conditions to the worker has been the historical definition. The AIHA Ergonomics Committee defines ergonomics as 'A multidisciplinary science that applies to principles based on the physical and psychological capabilities of people to the design or modification of jobs, equipment, products and work places'.
    Source: The Occupational Environment, Its Evaluation, Control, and Management. 3rd edition

2. Answer B.
    Explanation: WMSDs include a group of conditions that involve the nerves, tendons, and supporting structures, including the intervertebral discs. A wide range of disorders that can be mild, periodic, severe, chronic and debilitating.
    Source: The Occupational Environment, Its Evaluation, Control, and Management. 3rd edition

3. Answer C.
    Explanation: Chondromalacia, also called chondromalacia patellae, refers to softening and breakdown of the articular cartilage of the kneecap. Epicondylitis is an elbow condition, carpal tunnel is associated with the wrist, and adhesive capsulitis is a shoulder condition.
    Source: The Occupational Environment, Its Evaluation, Control, and Management. 3rd edition

4. Answer D.
    Explanation: Carpal Tunnel Syndrome is compression of the median nerve by the carpal ligament. Swelling of the tendon reduces the size of the tunnel under the ligament and pinches the nerve. Cubital Tunnel Syndrome is compression of the ulnar nerve below the elbow notch resulting in tingling, numbness, or pain in the ring and/or little finger. Pronator syndrome is caused by compression of the median nerve in the distal third of the forearm.
    Source: The Occupational Environment, Its Evaluation, Control, and Management. 3rd edition

5. Answer A.
    Explanation: Epicondylitis is an elbow condition (tennis elbow) associated with irritation of the tendons on the lateral portion of the elbow. Pronator syndrome is caused by compression of the median nerve in the distal third of the forearm. Raynaud's is also known as white finger syndrome.
    Source: The Occupational Environment, Its Evaluation, Control, and Management. 3rd edition

6. Answer D.
    Explanation: Neck Tension Syndrome is the condition associated with irritation/spasm of the levator scapulae and the trapezius muscle group, commonly occurring after prolonged overhead work. Thoracic outlet syndrome results from compression of the nerves and blood vessels between the clavicle and the first and second ribs at the brachial plexus. This limits blood flow to the arm resulting in numbness and weakness.
    Source: The Occupational Environment, Its Evaluation, Control, and Management. 3rd edition

7. Answer A.

    Explanation: Trigger finger is a type of tenosynovitis in which the tendon becomes locked or nearly locked so that forced movement is jerky. Raynaud's is also known as vibration syndrome and white finger syndrome.
    Source: The Occupational Environment, Its Evaluation, Control, and Management. 3rd edition

8. Answer B.

    Explanation: Repetition, force, low-temperature, static load, vibration, and posture are work-related risk factors for MSDs.
    Source: The Occupational Environment, Its Evaluation, Control, and Management. 3rd edition

9. Answer D.

    Explanation: Repetition, force, low-temperature, static load, vibration, and posture are work-related risk factors for MSDs.
    Source: The Occupational Environment, Its Evaluation, Control, and Management. 3rd edition

10. Answer D.

    Explanation: Repetition, force, low-temperature, static load, vibration, and posture are work-related risk factors for MSDs.
    Source: The Occupational Environment, Its Evaluation, Control, and Management. 3rd edition

11. Answer A.

    Explanation: Risk factors for the lower back include posture, frequency or repetition, static work, handles or coupling, asymmetrical handling, and space confinement.
    Source: The Occupational Environment, Its Evaluation, Control, and Management. 3rd edition

12. Answer D.

    Explanation: The physical work capacity, also known as aerobic capacity, is the maximum amount of oxygen that an individual can consume per minute. The greater the PWC for a task means that more physical stress and fatigue will occur.
    Source: The Occupational Environment, Its Evaluation, Control, and Management. 3rd edition

13. Answer D.

    Explanation: When lifting a load, it is important to do all of the following: securely grip the load, keep the load close to the body, use a comfortable posture, lift slowly and evenly, and do not twist the back.
    Source: NIOSH/CDC

14. Answer B.

    Explanation: The result of compression of the median nerve in the carpal tunnel of the wrist. The tunnel is an opening under the carpal ligament on the palmar side of the carpal bones. Through the tunnel passes the median nerve, the finger flexor tendons, and blood vessels. Swelling of the tendon sheaths reduce the size of the opening of the tunnel and pinch the median nerve and possibly blood vessels. The tunnel opening is also reduced if the wrist is flexed, extended or pivoted.
    Source: Fundamentals of Industrial Hygiene 5th Edition

---

15. Answer C.

Explanation: Cumulative strain injuries are the result of a series of micro-traumas, each of which can "insult" the body but not lead to discernible damage. In their accumulation over time, the micro-stresses can cause health complaints and result in disorders or injuries. Factors that are considered a significant importance of cumulative trauma disorders include awkward posture; high hand and finger forces; and high frequency or repetition.
Source: Fundamentals of Industrial Hygiene 5th Edition

16. Answer B.

Explanation: Ergonomics is the study of human characteristics for the design of the work environment. This knowledge may affect complex technical systems or work tasks, equipment, and workstations, or the tools and utensils used at work, at home, or during leisure times. Ergonomics is human- centered, transdisciplinary, and application-oriented.
Source: Fundamentals of Industrial Hygiene 5th Edition

17. Answer C.

Explanation: The use of lifting belts for professional material handling does not seem to be an effective way of preventing overexertion injuries. When lifting or lowering a load, humans instinctively develop intra-abdominal pressure within the trunk cavity. The pressure is believed to help support the curvature of the spine during the lifting or lowering effort. The back belt, or another external wrapping around the abdominal region, might help to maintain the internal pressure because it makes the walls of the pressure column stiffer. A large number of studies have been performed, summarized, and reviewed by McGill (1999), Lavender, et al (1998), and Thoumier, et al (1998) that neither support nor reject the wearing of support belts in industrial jobs.
Source: Fundamentals of Industrial Hygiene 5th Edition

18. Answer A.

Explanation: The 1991 NIOSH lifting equation is a specialized risk assessment tool. It has been designed to meet selected lifting related criteria and encompasses biomechanical, work physiology and psychophysical elements in a practical application framework that, if followed, will result in a reduced number of work place mishaps.

$$RWL = LC \times HM \times VM \times DM \times AM \times FM \times CM$$

$$RWL = 51\left(\tfrac{10}{H}\right)(1-.0075\,|\,V\text{-}30\,|)\left(.82+\tfrac{1.8}{D}\right)(1-(0.0032\times A))(FM)(CM)$$

$$RWL = 51\left(\tfrac{10}{24}\right)(1-.0075\times 6)\left(.82+\tfrac{1.8}{10}\right)(1-(0.0032 \times 15))(0.85)(0.9)$$

$$RWL = 51\times 0.417\times.955\times 1\times 0.952\times 0.85\times 0.9$$

$$RWL = 14.8\,lbs$$

19. Answer: B
    Explanation:

$$L\,I = \frac{L}{RWL}$$

$$L\,I = \frac{20}{14.8} = 1.35$$

The Lifting Index provides a numerical indicator of the need for redesign. An LI of greater than 1 indicates increased risk and above 3 requires corrective action. As noted in the previous question, this job could benefit from locating the work closer to the employee. Additionally, some value might be gained by shortening workday length devoted to lifting.

20. Answer D.
    Explanation:

$$RWL = LC \times HM \times VM \times DM \times AM \times FM \times CM$$

$$RWL(kg) = 23\left(\tfrac{25}{H}\right)(1 - .003\,|\,V - 75\,|)\left(.82 + \tfrac{4.5}{D}\right)\left(1 - (0.0032 \times A)\right)(FM)(CM)$$

$$RWL(kg) = 23\left(\tfrac{25}{45}\right)(1 - .003 \times 0)\left(.82 + \tfrac{4.5}{25}\right)\left(1 - (0.0032 \times 0)\right)(1)(1)$$

$$RWL(kg) = 23 \times 0.555 \times 1 \times 1 \times 1 \times 1 \times 1$$

$$RWL(kg) = 12.77\,kg$$

Rubric 9: Health Risk Analysis and Hazard Communication

Familiarity and proper application of the principles of health risk analysis and hazard communication is an important function for the occupational/industrial hygiene professional. This includes the use and interpretation of the ACGIH Threshold Limit Value, Biological Exposure Indices, and industrial ventilation publications. In addition, the professional must be knowledgeable about the guidelines published by the American National Standards Institute (ANSI), the American Society for Heating, Refrigeration, and Air Conditioning Engineers (AHRAE), and the National Institute for Occupational Safety and Health (NIOSH).

Control Banding

Control banding (CB) originally appeared in the 1990s in response to the following factors: numerous new chemicals that were threats to worker health; legal challenges to developing regulatory standards; the lack of resources (and effort) to conduct toxicological and epidemiological research needed to establish the OELs; and developing analytical methods for exposure monitoring.

Control banding is a qualitative or semi-quantitative approach to risk management and risk assessment. Control measures are developed for a specific chemical based on the chemical's hazard classification, the amount of chemical being used, and the chemicals volatility/dustiness. Once the chemical has been placed in the correct "band" of control measures, the consequence is a recommended control strategy for that specific chemical.

Control of Substances Hazardous to Health (COSHH) Essentials is a heavily used control banding approach developed by the Health and Safety Executive (HSE) in the United Kingdom. It was put in place to assist employers in meeting the requirements of the COSHH regulations to conduct risk assessments of chemical exposures to workers. The goal of COSHH Essentials is to determine a recommended level of control approach by combining the hazard with the exposure potential. The assessment of the hazard and the exposure potential is meant to guide toward one of the four risk management approaches: (1) general ventilation; (2) engineering controls; (3) containment; or (4) special controls. To assist non-expert users of COSHH Essentials in implementing the levels of control, over 300 control guidance sheets (CGS) have been developed to provide general and specific advice on a range of hazards, tasks, and worker protection topics (Health and Safety Executive, 2009).

Even though COSHH Essentials is the most pronounced control banding approach, other control banding approaches have been developed and utilized in the Occupational Safety and Health field.

As with any approach, there are critics of CB. The American Conference of Governmental Industrial Hygienists criticized CB for being too simple and relying on limited data.
Source: The Occupational Environment: Its Evaluation, Control and Management, 3ʳᵈ Edition

Hazard Communication

A systematically developed comprehensive safety and health management program is the most beneficial approach to worker safety and health in a workplace. A direct foundation to this approach is efficient and effective communication of hazardous materials in the workplace. Lack of information about the chemicals in use makes it very difficult for an occupational hygienist to design and implement an appropriate protective program for employees exposed to chemicals in the workplace. A key objective for any hazardous communication **program** is to provide information to employees and safety professionals, and empower employees to be active participants in an employer's safety and health program. The goal of a hazardous communication program is to reduce the potential for chemical source illnesses and injuries by providing transparent and effective communication to all employers and employees about the potential chemical hazards in the workplace.

If an employer has hazardous chemicals in the workplace, then the workplace must have a written hazardous communication program. For example, hazardous chemicals stored in containers must be labeled, a Safety Data Sheet (SDS) must be available for each hazardous chemical in the workplace, and training employees on hazards, and how to obtain and translate the hazard information, is a necessity. Like any safety program, modification and refining is essential. OSHA implemented a Global Harmonized System (GHS) for classification and labeling of chemicals in order to incorporate more detailed specifications for hazard classification and labeling in the Hazard Communication Standard (HCS). These modifications attempt to increase the clarity of information provided to workers, which can lead to additional reductions in chemical source illness and injuries in the workplace.
Source: The Occupational Environment: Its Evaluation, Control and Management, 3rd Edition

Hierarchy of Controls

According to American National Standard Institute, Occupational Health and Safety Management System, hierarchy of controls intends to provide a systematic approach to eliminate, reduce, or control the risk of different hazards. Each step is considered less effective than the one before it. It is not unusual to combine several steps to achieve an acceptable risk. Things to consider in detraining methods of hazard elimination or control include types of hazards employees are exposed to, the severity of the hazards, and the risk the hazards pose to employees. See the Hierarchy of Health and Safety Controls based on ANSI z-10 below.

CONTROLS	EXAMPLES
1. Elimination	Design to eliminate hazards: falls, HAZMAT, confined spaces, materials handling, tools and machinery, etc.
2. Substitution	Substitute for less hazardous materials and equipment, reduce energy, etc.
3. Engineering Controls	Incorporate safety trough design, such as ventilation systems, enclosures, guarding, interlocks, lift tables, conveyors, etc.
4. Warnings	Strategically place signs, alarms, enunciators, labels, etc.
5. Administrative Controls	Standard Operating Procedures (SOPs) such as: Conduct JSAs, job rotation, inspections, training, mentoring, etc.
6. Personal Protective Equipment	PPE assessments may result in the use of safety glasses, goggles, face shields, fall protection, protective footwear, gloves, respirators, chemical suits, etc.

Risk Reduction

According to the World Health Organization, risk reduction involves measures designed either to prevent hazards from creating risks or to lessen the distribution, intensity or severity of hazards.
Source: World Health Organization (WHO) Risk Reduction and Emergency Preparedness

According to ACGIH, the Threshold Limit Values (TLVs) are guidelines to be used by professional hygienist. The values are guidelines or recommendations, not regulations. They can assist with the evaluation and control of potential workplace health hazards. TLVs refer to airborne concentrations of chemical substances and represent conditions under which it is believed that nearly all workers may be repeatedly exposed over a working lifetime, without adverse health effects.

Threshold Limit Value – Time-Weighted Average (TLV-TWA)
According to ACGIH, the TLV-TWA is the TWA concentration for a conventional 8-hour workday and a 40-hour workweek, to which it is believed that nearly all workers may be repeatedly exposed for a working lifetime without adverse effect.

*Threshold Limit Value – Short-Term Exposure Limit (TLV-STEL)*According to ACGIH, the TLV-STEL is a 15-minute TWA exposure that should not be exceeded at any time during a work day, even if the 8-hour TWA is within the TLV-TWA. The TLV-STEL is the concentration to which it is believed that workers can be exposed continuously for a short period of time without suffering from 1) irritation, 2) chronic or irreversible tissue damage, 3) dose-related toxic effects, or 4) narcosis of sufficient degree to increase the likelihood of accidental injury, impaired self-rescue, or materially reduced work efficiency.

Threshold Limit Value – Ceiling (TLV-C)
According to ACGIH, the TLV-C is the concentration that should not be exceeded during any part of the working exposure. If instantaneous measurements are not available, sampling should be conducted for the minimum period of time sufficient to detect exposures at or above the ceiling value.
Source: ACGIH TLVs and BEIs Based on the Documentation of the Threshold Limit Values for Chemical Substances and Physical Agents & Biological Exposure Indices

Calculating Time Weighted Average - TWA

$$TWA = \frac{(C_1 \times T_1) + (C_2 \times T_2) + \cdots + (C_n \times T_n)}{(T_1 + T_2 + \cdots + T_n)}$$

Where C_1 is the measured concentration for a corresponding time period.

$T_{1\ldots}$ is the time period for a corresponding sample period concentration.

Note: Time units must be consistent (either all minutes or all hours).

Use:

To determine an 8-hour or full period time weighted average when short duration samples were obtained.

Example:

Calculate the 8-hour time weighted average for the following toluene exposure monitoring data.

Sample Identification	Sample Duration	Analytical Results
Sample 1 A	200 minutes	55 parts per million
Sample 1 B	180 minutes	70 parts per million
Sample 1 C	100 minutes	200 parts per million

$$TWA = \frac{(C_1 x T_1) + (C_2 x T_2) + \cdots + (C_n x T_n)}{(T_1 + T_2 + \cdots + T_n)}$$

$$TWA = \frac{(55 ppm x 200 min) + (70 ppm x 180 min) + (200 ppm x 100 min)}{(200\ min + 180 min + 100 min)}$$

$$TWA = 90.8 \text{ ppm}$$
(note: 8-hours = 480 minutes)

Calculating the TLV for a Mixture of Chemicals in Air with Additive Health Effects

$$TLV_{mix} = \frac{C_1}{TLV_1} + \frac{C_2}{TLV_2} + \frac{C_n}{TLV_n} \cdots$$

Where:

TLV_{mix} is the Threshold Limit Value for a mixture of airborne chemicals with additive effects. If the sum is greater than one (1), then an overexposure exists.

C_1 is the measured concentration of chemical 1 in air.

C_n is the measured concentration of chemical n in air.

TLV_1 is the published Threshold Limit Value for the chemical 1.

$TLVn$ is the published Threshold Limit Value for chemical n.

Use:

When two or more hazardous chemicals with similar toxic effects are present in the environment, the combined effect should be evaluated, rather than the individual effect. *Note*: The units can be either mg/m^3 or ppm, but must be consistent in the equation.

Example:

A worker was exposed to the following chemicals in air: Hexane at 30 ppm, Toluene at 16 ppm, and xylene at 40 ppm. Does the exposure exceed the 8-hour time weighted average? The TLVs for each are hexane 50 ppm, toluene 20 ppm and xylene 100 ppm.

$$TLV_{mix} = \frac{C_1}{TLV_1} + \frac{C_2}{TLV_2} + \frac{C_n}{TLV_n}$$

$$TLV_{mix} = \frac{30}{50} + \frac{16}{20} + \frac{40}{100}$$

$$TLV_{mix} = 1.8$$

1.8 is greater than unity (1) and therefore an overexposure.

Calculating the TLV for a Mixture of Vapors in Air from a Liquid

$$TLV_{mix} = \cfrac{1}{\cfrac{f_1}{TLV_1} + \cfrac{f_2}{TLV_2} + \cfrac{f_n}{TLV_n}}$$

Where:

TLV_{mix} is the Threshold Limit Value for a mixture of chemicals based on evaporation of liquids into vapor in air.

f_1 is the fractional weight in percent of chemical 1 in the liquid mixture expressed in decimal form.

f_n is the fractional weight in percent of chemical n in the liquid mixture expressed in decimal form.

TLV_1 is the Threshold Limit Value of chemical 1 in the mixture.

Use:

Calculate an exposure limit for a mixture when the liquid mixture percentages are known (data sheets, labels, etc.) and that the health effects are additive. Useful for setting an alarm on a direct reading device. *Note*: The formula assumes the liquids evaporate equally into the atmosphere. Mass fraction requires the TLV are in mass/volume units.

Example:

A review of the data sheet for a cleaning solution reveals the following: Toluene 20%, Xylene 40%, and Hexane 40%. The TLV book lists the TLV for Toluene as 188 mg/m^3, Xylene as 434 mg/m^3, and Hexane as 176 mg/m^3 (or you may have to convert from ppm to mg/m^3). Calculate TLV_{mix} to use as the alarm point for the vapor detection device.

$$TLV_{mix} = \cfrac{1}{\cfrac{f_1}{TLV_1} + \cfrac{f_2}{TLV_2} + \cfrac{f_n}{TLV_n}}$$

$$TLV_{mix} = \cfrac{1}{\cfrac{.20}{188\frac{mg}{m3}} + \cfrac{.40}{434\frac{mg}{m3}} + \cfrac{.40}{176\frac{mg}{m3}}}$$

$$TLV_{mix} = 239\frac{mg}{m3}$$

Brief and Scala Method

The Brief and Scala (1975) method is regarded as the most conservative model and considers the impact of the number of increased hours worked and the recovery time between exposure periods. No consideration of the agent's activity in the body is made. Using either the daily or weekly equation detailed below, a reduction factor is determined and then applied to the TWA exposure standard

Brief & Scala Alternate Shift Length Reduction Factor

$$RF = \frac{8}{h} x \frac{24 - h}{16}$$

Where:
RF is the reduction factor for extended shifts (no units)
h is the number of hours worked per shift
Note: 24 - h represents the exposure-free hours per day

Use:
Calculating a reduction factor for alternate work shifts that are greater than 8-hours in a single day.

Example:
Calculate the daily exposure reduction factor for a worker who works 10-hour shifts.

$$RF = \frac{8}{h} x \frac{24 - h}{16}$$

Step 1: Insert the length of the shift in hours into the formula

$$RF = \frac{8}{10} x \frac{24 - 10}{16}$$

$$RF = 0.7$$

Note: To obtain the revised exposure limit, multiply the reduction factor by exposure limit.

Brief & Scala Alternate Work Week Reduction Factor

$$RF = \frac{40}{h_w} x \frac{168 - h_w}{128}$$

Where:
RF is the reduction factor (no unit)
h_w is the hours worked in one week
Note: $168 - h_w$ represents the exposure-free hours per week

Use:
Calculating a reduction factor for alternate work weeks that are greater than 8-hours per day, 5-days per week.

Example:
The published exposure limit is 100 ppm as an 8-hour TWA. What is the adjusted exposure limit for workers who are consistently working seven (7) days per week?

Step 1: Calculate the reduction factor 8 hours/day x 7 days/week

$$RF = \frac{40}{h_w} x \frac{168 - h_w}{128}$$

$$RF = \frac{40}{56} x \frac{168 - 56}{128}$$

$$RF = 0.625$$

Step 2: Calculate the adjusted exposure limit

$$\text{Adjusted Exposure Limit} = 0.625 \text{ x } 100 \text{ ppm}$$

$$\text{Adjusted Exposure Limit} = 62.5 \text{ ppm}$$

Airborne Concentration Using Fiber Density (E)

$$C_{asb} = \frac{EA_c}{(V_s)(10^3)}$$

Where:

C_{asb} is the concentration of fibers in air, expressed as fibers/mL

E is the fiber density as measured on the filter, expressed as fibers/mm^2

A_c is the effective fiber collection area of a filter, typically expressed as 385 mm^2 for a 25 mm filter

V is the volume of sampled air in liters

Use:

To determine the airborne fiber concentration in fibers/mL which is equivalent to fibers/cc.

Example:

The microscopy technician has analyzed a filter for asbestos and determined that the fiber density is 381 f/mm^2. The duration of sampling was 450 minutes. The pump was pre-calibrated at 2 L/m and the flow rate was verified at 2.0 L/m after sampling. The effective collection area of a filter is approximately 385 mm^2 for a 25 mm filter. Calculate the airborne concentration.

$$C_{asb} = \frac{EA_c}{(V_s)(10^3)}$$

Step 1: Calculate the volume of air sampled

$$450 \text{ minutes x 2 L/m} = 900L$$

Step 2: Solve for C_{asb}

$$C_{asb} = \frac{(381\frac{f}{mm^2})(385mm^2)}{(900L)(10^3\frac{mL}{L})}$$

C_{asb} = 0.16 f/mL and since mL and cc are equivalent 0.16 f/cc

Airborne Concentration of Fibers with the Fiber Density Calculation in the Numerator

$$C_{asb} = \frac{(C_s - C_b)A_c}{1000\,(A_f)(V_s)}$$

Where:

C_{asb} is the concentration of fibers in air, expressed as fibers per ml (f/ml)

C_s is the average number of fibers counted on the **sample** cassette filter per graticule field

C_b is the average number of fibers counted on the **blank** cassette filter per graticule field

V_s is the volume of sampled air in liters

A_f is the area of the graticule field – roughly 0.00785 mm^2

A_c is the effective fiber collection area of a filter, typically expressed as 385 mm^2 for a 25 mm filter

Use:

To calculate the airborne concentration of fibers with the fiber density calculation in the numerator

Example:

An IH trained in phase contrast microscopy is analyzing a filter for airborne asbestos fiber concentration. The sample for asbestos was collected over 450 minutes of an 8-hour shift at 2 L/m. After counting 100 fields, the average fiber count is 3 fibers per field. The field blank contains 0.01 fibers per field. It is known that the area of a 25 mm filter is 385 mm^2 and that the area of a graticule field is approximately 0.00785 mm^2. What is the fiber concentration, and is the sample acceptable?

Step 1: Calculate the volume of air sampled

$$450 \text{ minutes x 2 L/m} = 900L$$

Step 2: Solve for C_{asb}

$$C_{asb} = \frac{(C_s - C_b)A_c}{1000\,(A_f)(V_s)}$$

$$C_{asb} = \frac{(3 - 0.01\ fibers)385mm^2}{1000\dfrac{mL}{L}\,(0.00785mm^2)(900\ L)}$$

C_{asb} = 0.16 f/mL and since mL and cc are equivalent 0.16 f/cc

The PEL for asbestos is 0.1 f/cc

Source: NIOSH Manual of Analytical Methods

Fiber Density Calculation

$$E_{fiber\ density} = \frac{\dfrac{F}{N_f} - \dfrac{B}{N_b}}{A_f}$$

Where:

$E_{fiber\ density}$ is amount of fibers on the sample filter, expressed as fibers/mm²

f/N_f is the average or mean fiber count per graticule field

B/N_b is the mean fiber count per graticule field of the blank filter

A_f is the graticule field area - roughly 0.00785 mm²

Use:

The first step in determining airborne fiber concentration.

Note: Fiber density > 1300 f/mm² are reported as uncountable or probably biased.

Example:

An IH technician trained in phase contrast microscopy is analyzing a filter for asbestos fiber density on the filter. Calculating the fiber density is the first of a two-step method for determining the airborne fiber concentration. If the fiber density is greater than 1300 f/mm², the results are reported as uncountable or probably biased. The sample for asbestos was collected over 450 minutes of an 8-hour shift at 2 L/m. After counting 100 fields, the average fiber count is 3 fibers per field. The field blank contains 0.01 fibers per field. It is known that the area of a 25 mm filter is 385 mm² and that the area of a graticule field is approximately 0.00785 mm². What is the fiber density, and is the sample acceptable?

Step 1: Calculate and report fiber density on the filter, E (fibers/mm²):

$$E_{fiber\ density} = \frac{\dfrac{F}{N_f} - \dfrac{B}{N_b}}{A_f}$$

$$E_{fiber\ density} = \frac{3 - 0.01\ fibers}{0.00785\ mm^2}$$

$$E_{fiber\ density} = 381\ f/mm2$$

Note: Fiber counts above 1300 fibers/mm² and fiber counts from samples with >50% of filter area covered with particulate should be reported as "uncountable" or "probably biased." Other fiber counts outside the 100–1300 fiber/mm² range should be reported as having "greater than optimal variability" and as being "probably biased." *NIOSH 7400*

Microscopic Limit of Resolution

$$d = \frac{0.61\lambda}{\eta \sin\alpha}$$

Where:

d is distance. It is the shortest distance between two lines that can be observed by an optical microscope

λ is the light wavelength, expressed as nanometers

η is the index of refraction for the material between the specimen and the lens depending on the technique (oil immersion, air, etc.)

α is the half angle

Use:

To determine the resolution or level of detail that can be viewed through the microscope lens.

Note: The index of refraction for air is 1.0, water is 1.33 and oil is 1.52.

Based on this equation, NIOSH 7400 PCM can view fibers that are approximately 0.2μm and larger in diameter.

Example:

An optical microscope is used with the following conditions. Violet light (400 nm) is used to observe a sample in air. The sin of α for this microscope is 0.95. Calculate the theoretical limit of resolution.

Step 1: Solve for d

$$d = \frac{0.61\lambda}{\eta \sin\alpha}$$

$$d = \frac{0.61 \; x \; 400nm}{1.0 \; x \; 0.95}$$

$$d = 257 \text{ nm or } 0.26 \text{ μm}$$

Rubric 9: Health Risk Analysis and Hazard Communication Questions

1. When conducting sampling for the alcohol Cyclohexanol, what is the recommended media?

    A) Solid Sorbent tube.
    B) 1 μm PTFE filter.
    C) 5 μm Preweighed PVC filter.
    D) Silica Gel Tube.

2. What is the appropriate method when sampling for Vinyl Chloride?

    A) NIOSH 1007.
    B) NIOSH 1200.
    C) NIOSH 1300.
    D) NIOSH 1301.

3. What is the appropriate method and recommended media when sampling for Methene Chloride (Dichloromethane)?

    A) NIOSH 1000; Solid Sorbent Tube.
    B) NIOSH 1005; Silica Gel Tube.
    C) NIOSH 1000; Silica Gel Tube.
    D) NIOSH 1005; Solid Sorbent Tube.

4. Which of the following is not a category of Occupational Exposure Limits (OELs)?

    A) Regulatory Standard (OSHA).
    B) Voluntary Guidelines (ACGIH).
    C) Regional Standards.
    D) Local Limits (e.g., Company Limits).

5. A qualitative evaluation is a walk-through inspection that identifies which of the following hazards?

    A) Visual and Auditory.
    B) Olfactory and Irritant.
    C) Visual, Auditory, and Olfactory.
    D) Olfactory, Irritant, and Auditory.

6. Choose the statement that is not associated with risk communication.
    A) Risk communication shall be implemented only at the highest level of management to eliminate possible confusion.
    B) Risk communication exchanges information and opinions pertaining to a hazard, the hazards magnitude and significance, and potential control methods.
    C) Risk communication strives to lessen the tension in a situation by communicating in a way that everyone involved can comprehend.
    D) Risk communication is the exchange of information and opinions among parties.

7. The risk management process usually follows a general systematic order. The five steps are:

    1. Implementing controls.
    2. Identifying hazards.
    3. Supervising and evaluating.
    4. Developing controls and making risk decisions.
    5. Assessing hazards to determine risk.

<u>What is the correct **numerical order** of the five erisk management processes listed above?</u>

    A) 2, 5, 4, 1, 3
    B) 1, 5, 4, 2, 3
    C) 3, 2, 1, 5, 4
    D) 5, 1, 4, 3,2

8. If it can be reasonable to conclude that the chemicals present in the workplace could add, one on the other, to the total effect, then it is also reasonable to consider adding the exposure assessment to derive a total exposure assessment. An example would be the presence of three chemicals, X, Y, and Z, each having a similar toxicological effect on the same target organ. The total value (TV) is determined based on the concentration (C) and the threshold limit value (TLV) of each of the chemicals using the following equation:

$$TV = \frac{C_1}{TLV_1} + \frac{C_2}{TLV_2} + \cdots + \frac{C_n}{TLV_n}$$

Assume 30 ppm of acetone with a TLV of 250 ppm; 10 pm of toluene with a TLV of 20 ppm; and 110 ppm, of 2-propanol with a TLV of 200 ppm. Calculate the total value (TV).

    A) 0.40
    B) 0.74
    C) 1.17
    D) 1.46

9. Choose the statement that best describes the Implementation and Operation Component of the ISO 14000 Series.

   A) Develop an environmental policy that includes commitment to improvement and pollution prevention; commitment to comply with regulations; provides a framework for environmental objective setting and review; and is made available to the public.
   B) Includes procedures to ensure that environmental concerns are properly planned for, addresses strategies to prevent significant environmental impacts through the use of legal strategies, and objective and goal setting.
   C) Addresses the establishment of clearly defined roles and responsibilities. Sufficient resources will be allocated to ensure environmental program effectiveness. Top management commitment will be necessitated to support environmental policy requirements. Key environmental training and awareness needs will be identified and addressed.
   D) Protocols will be developed and implemented to evaluate adherence to environmental standards and good management practices.

10. Which of the following categories of carcinogenicity represents the "Suspected Human Carcinogen" carcinogenicity category?

    A) A1
    B) A2
    C) A3
    D) A4
    E) A5

11. Who generates the TLVs and BEIs Handbook?

    A) American Center of Governmental Industrial Hygienist.
    B) Occupational Safety and Health Administration (OSHA).
    C) Board of Certified Safety Professionals (BCSP).
    D) American Conference of Governmental Industrial Hygienist.

12. Choose the statement that best describes a TLV-short-term exposure limit (STEL).

    A) The threshold limit value-short term exposure limit (TLV-STEL) is the concentration to which it is believed that workers can be exposed continuously for a 30-minute, time-weighted average exposure and should not be exceeded at any time during a workday, even if the 8-hour time-weighted average is within the TLV-TWA.

    B) The threshold limit value-shift total exposure limit (TLV-STEL) is the concentration to which it is believed that workers can be exposed continuously for a 30-minute, total-weighted average exposure and should not be exceeded at any time during a workday, even if the 4-hour total-weighted average is within the TLV-TWA.

    C) The threshold limit value-short term exposure limit (TLV-STEL) is the concentration to which it is believed that workers can be exposed continuously for a 15-minute, time-weighted average exposure and should not be exceeded at any time during a workday, even if the 8-hour time-weighted average is within the TLV-TWA.

    D) A threshold limit value that provides a short-term baseline limit for all aerosols and particulates is found in the TLV & BEI Handbook.

13. When is it necessary to apply an excursion limit?

    A) There is a TLV-TWA and no TLV-STEL regardless of the 8-hour TLV-TWA limit.
    B) There is no TLV-TWA or TLV-STEL.
    C) There is no TLV-TWA regardless of the TLV-STEL limit.
    D) There is a TLV-TWA and a TLV-STEL.

14. Why is it important to limit short term exposures at high concentrations?

    A) Prevent rapidly occurring adverse health effects.
    B) Prevent chronic adverse health effects.
    C) Prevent rapidly occurring and chronic adverse health effects.
    D) To maintain baseline data for the short term high exposure.

15. Convert 10 ppm of Methylene chloride to milligrams per cubic meter. Reference information includes:

- Methylene chloride: CH_2Cl_2
- Atomic Mass: C = 12, H = 1 & Cl = 35.5

    A) 11.9
    B) 20.5
    C) 34.7
    D) 70.5

16. An industrial hygienist conducted an 8-hour TWA sampling for acetone, ethyl acetate, and ethyl ether. See concentrations below:

   - Acetone: 500 ppm
   - Ethyl Acetate: 100 ppm
   - Ethyl Ether: 110 ppm

   Acetone's 8-hour TWA Permissible Exposure Limit (PEL) is 1,000 ppm. Ethyl Acetate's 8-hour TWA Permissible Exposure Limit (PEL) is 400 ppm. Ethyl Ether's 8-hour TWA Permissible Exposure Limit (PEL) is 400 ppm. What is the additive mixture exposure value for acetone, ethyl acetate, and ethyl ether? Does this value make the worker overexposed?

   A) 0.15, the worker is not overexposed.
   B) 0.88, the worker is not overexposed.
   C) 1.025, the worker is overexposed.
   D) 1.80, the worker is overexposed.

17. When testing for chromium (VI) using the Biological Exposure Indices (BEIs), what determinate do you test for?

   A) Chromium in the urine.
   B) Chromium in the blood.
   C) Cadmium in the urine.
   D) Cadmium in the blood.

18. When testing for toluene using the Biological Exposure Indices (BEIs), when should you conduct sampling for the determinant?

   A) Toluene in blood → prior to the last shift of the work week; Toluene in urine → at the end of a shift.
   B) Toluene in urine → prior to the last shift of the work week; Toluene in blood → at the end of a shift.
   C) Toluene in blood → at the end of a shift; Toluene in urine → at the end of a shift.
   D) Toluene in blood → prior to the last shift of the work week; Toluene in urine → prior to the last shift of the work week.

19. Calculate the weekly exposure reduction factor for a worker who works 8-hour shifts, seven days a week.

   A) 0.24
   B) 0.44
   C) 0.63
   D) 0.76

20. An optical microscope is being used with the following conditions. The light source has a specified wavelength of 450 nm. The slide is being viewed through water. The desired limit of resolution is 0.20 μm. According to the literature, the sine of an angle for this microscope is 0.97. Calculate the theoretical limit of resolution.

    A) 0.20 μm
    B) 2.0 μm
    C) 210 μm
    D) 213 nm

Rubric 9: Health Risk Analysis and Hazard Communication Answers

1. Answer A.
   Explanation: According to the NIOSH Manual of Analytical Methods, method 1402, the recommended media when sampling for Cyclohexanol is a solid sorbent tube (coconut shell). The analysis is done via gas chromatography-FID.
   Source: NIOSH Manual of Analytical Methods 4th edition

2. Answer A.
   Explanation: According to the NIOSH Manual of Analytical Methods, the appropriate method when sampling for Vinyl Chloride is NIOSH 1007. Method 1007 specifies solid sorbent tubes (2 – tandem) and analysis by gas chromatography + FID.
   Source: NIOSH Manual of Analytical Methods 4th edition

3. Answer D.
   Explanation: According to the NIOSH Manual of Analytical Methods, the appropriate method when sampling for Methylene Chloride is NIOSH 1005. According to the NIOSH Manual of Analytical Methods, the recommended media when sampling for Methylene Chloride is two solid sorbent tubes (coconut shell) in sequence. The sample is analyzed with gas chromatography-FID. An electron capture device (ECD) may also be used to achieve a lower detection level.
   Source: NIOSH Manual of Analytical Methods 4th edition

4. Answer C.
   Explanation: The three categories of Occupational Exposure Limits (OELs) are regulatory standards, voluntary guidelines, and local limits.
   Source: The Occupational Environment: Its Evaluation, Control and Management 3rd edition, Volume 1

5. Answer C.
   Explanation: Evaluation is the process of examining an operation to determine the extent to which health hazards are present. Qualitative evaluations identify visual, auditory, and olfactory hazards when going through a walk-through inspection.
   Source: The Occupational Environment: Its Evaluation, Control and Management 3rd edition, Volume 1

6. Answer A.
   Explanation: Risk communication is the exchange of information and opinions among parties. Risk communication exchanges information pertaining to a hazard, the hazard's magnitude and significance, and potential control methods. Risk communication strives to lessen the tension in a situation by communicating in a way that everyone involved can comprehend.
   Source: The Occupational Environment: Its Evaluation, Control and Management 3rd edition, Volume 1

7. Answer A.
   Explanation:
   1. Identifying hazards
   2. Assessing hazards to determine risk
   3. Developing controls and making risk decisions
   4. Implementing controls
   5. Supervising and evaluating

   Source: The Occupational Environment: Its Evaluation, Control and Management 3rd edition, Volume 1

8. Answer C.
   Explanation:

$$TV = \frac{C_1}{TLV_1} + \frac{C_2}{TLV_2} + \cdots + \frac{C_n}{TLV_n}$$

Assume 30 ppm of acetone with a TLV of 250 ppm; 10 pm of toluene with a TLV of 20 ppm; and 110 ppm, of 2-propanol with a TLV of 200 ppm. Calculate the total value (TV).

Step 1: Solve for TV

$$TV = \frac{C_1}{TLV_1} + \frac{C_2}{TLV_2} + \cdots + \frac{C_n}{TLV_n}$$

$$TV = \frac{30}{250} + \frac{10}{20} + \frac{110}{200}$$

$$TV = 0.12 + 0.5 + 0.55$$

$$TV = 1.17$$

The general standard for the total value is 1.00. It could be judged from this evaluation that the exposure may have an additive impact above acceptable limits, and the exposure should be reduced. *Source: The Occupational Environment: Its Evaluation, Control and Management 3rd edition, Volume 1*

9. Answer C.
    Explanation:
    Components of ISO 14000

Environmental Policy	Develop an environmental policy that includes commitment to improvement and pollution prevention. It should also contain a commitment to comply with regulations and provide a framework for objective setting and review. It must be documented, implemented, and communicated to all employees and made available to the public.
Planning	Includes procedures to ensure that plans are developed to address environmental concerns. The plans should prevent significant environmental impacts through the use of legal strategies and goal setting. Written programs must be established for all relevant environmental areas.
Implementation and Operation	ISO 14001 addresses the establishment of defined roles and responsibilities. Sufficient resources must be allocated to ensure environmental program effectiveness. Top management commitment is required. Key environmental training and awareness needs will be identified and addressed.
Checking and Corrective Action	Protocols will be developed and implemented. Adherence to environmental standards and good management practices must be evaluated. Corrective action procedures must be developed and used.
Management Review	Periodic reviews must be conducted by top management to ensure the management system adequately addresses environmental concerns and compliance.

10. Answer B.
    Explanation: The categories of carcinogenicity are:
    - **A1**- Confirmed Human Carcinogen: The agent is carcinogenic to humans based on the weight of the evidence from epidemiologic studies.
    - **A2**- Suspected Human Carcinogen: Human data is accepted as adequate in quality but are conflicting or insufficient to classify the agent as a confirmed human carcinogen; OR, the agent is carcinogenic in experimental animals at dose(s), by route(s) of exposure, at site(s) of histologic type(s), or by mechanism(s) considered relevant to worker exposure.
    - **A3**- Confirmed Animal Carcinogen with Unknown Relevance to Humans: The agent is carcinogenic in experimental animals at a relatively high dose, by route(s) of administration, at site(s) of histologic type(s), or by mechanism(s) that may not be relevant to worker exposure.
    - **A4**- Not Classifiable as a Human Carcinogen: Agents which cause concern that they could be carcinogenic for humans, but which cannot be assessed conclusively because of lack of data. In vitro or animal studies do not provide indications of carcinogenicity that are sufficient to classify the agent into one or the other categories.

- **A5**- Not Suspected as a Human Carcinogen: The agent is not suspected to be a human carcinogen on the basis of properly conducted epidemiologic studies in humans.
  Source: TLVs and BEIS Based on the Documentation of the Threshold Limit Values for Chemical Substances and Physical Agents & Biological Exposure Indices

11. Answer D.
    Explanation: The American Conference of Governmental Industrial Hygienist is a member based organization that generates an annual updated version of the TLVs and BEIs handbook.
    Source: TLVs and BEIS Based on the Documentation of the Threshold Limit Values for Chemical Substances and Physical Agents & Biological Exposure Indices

12. Answer C.
    Explanation: A 15-minute TWA exposure that should not be exceeded at any time during a workday, even if the 8-hour TWA is within the TLV-TWA. The TLV-STEL is the concentration to which it is believed that workers can be exposed continuously for a short period of time without suffering from 1) irritation, 2) chronic or irreversible tissue damage, 3) dose-rate-dependent toxic effects, or 4) narcosis of sufficient degree to increase the likelihood of accidental injury, impaired self-rescue, or materially reduced work efficiency. The TLV-STEL will not necessarily protect against these effects if the daily TLV-TWA is exceeded. *Source: TLVs and BEIS Based on the Documentation of the Threshold Limit Values for Chemical Substances and Physical Agents & Biological Exposure Indices*

13. Answer A.
    Explanation: For many substances with a TLV-TWA, there is no TLV-STEL. Nevertheless, excursions above the TLV-TWA should be controlled, even where the 8-hour TLV-TWA is within recommended limits. Excursion limits apply to those TLV-TWAs that do not have TLV-STELs.
    Source: TLVs and BEIS Based on the Documentation of the Threshold Limit Values for Chemical Substances and Physical Agents & Biological Exposure Indices

14. Answer D.
    Explanation: Short-term peak exposures above the TLV-TWA should be controlled, even where the 8-hour TLV-TWA is within recommended limits. Limiting short-term high exposures is intended to prevent rapidly occurring acute adverse health effects resulting from transient peak exposures during a work shift. Since these adverse effects may occur at some multiple of the 8-hour TWA, even if they have not yet been documented, it is prudent to limit peak exposures.
    Source: TLVs and BEIS Based on the Documentation of the Threshold Limit Values for Chemical Substances and Physical Agents & Biological Exposure Indices

15. Answer C.

    Explanation:

    Conversion from ppm to $\frac{mg}{m^3}$.

    $$\frac{mg}{m^3} = \frac{(ppm)(gram\ molecular\ weight\ of\ substance)}{24.45}$$

    Where 24.45 = molar volume of air in liters at NTP conditions (25°C and 760 torr) and Molecular Weight = $\frac{g}{mol}$

    $$\frac{mg}{m^3} = \frac{(ppm)(gram\ molecular\ weight\ of\ substance)}{24.45}$$

    $$\frac{mg}{m^3} = \frac{(10ppm)(84.9\frac{g}{mol})}{24.45}$$

    $$\frac{mg}{m^3} = 34.7$$

    Source: TLVs and BEIS Based on the Documentation of the Threshold Limit Values for Chemical Substances and Physical Agents & Biological Exposure Indices

16. Answer C.

    Explanation:

    Step 1: Use the Additive Mixture Formula

    $$\frac{C_1}{T_1} + \frac{C_2}{T_2} \cdots \frac{C_n}{T_n}$$

    $$\frac{500\ ppm}{1,000\ ppm} + \frac{100\ ppm}{400\ ppm} + \frac{110\ ppm}{400\ ppm} = .50 + .25 + .275 = 1.025$$

    Since the unity is greater than 1.0, the worker is overexposed due to the additive mixture effect.

    Source: TLVs and BEIS Based on the Documentation of the Threshold Limit Values for Chemical Substances and Physical Agents & Biological Exposure Indices

17. Answer A.

    Explanation: The test for Chromium (VI) is for the total chromium in the urine to be conducted at the end of a shift at the end of the workweek.

    Source: TLVs and BEIS Based on the Documentation of the Threshold Limit Values for Chemical Substances and Physical Agents & Biological Exposure Indices

18. Answer A.
    Explanation: The test for toluene is for the toluene in the blood and in the urine. If you test for toluene in the blood, you should conduct sampling for the determinant prior to the last shift of the workweek. If you test for toluene in the urine, you should conduct sampling for the determinant at the end of a shift.
    Source: TLVs and BEIS Based on the Documentation of the Threshold Limit Values for Chemical Substances and Physical Agents & Biological Exposure Indices

19. Answer C.
    Explanation: Using the Brief and Scala reduction for extended work weeks and the shift is 8-hours per day, calculate the reduction factor.

$$RF = \frac{40}{h_w} \; x \; \frac{168 - h_w}{128}$$

$$RF = \frac{40}{56} \; x \; \frac{168 - 56}{128}$$

$$RF = 0.71 \; x \; 0.875$$

$$RF = 0.625 \; or \; 0.63$$

20. Answer D.
    Explanation:
    Step 1: Solve for d

$$d = \frac{0.61\lambda}{\eta sin\alpha}$$

$$d = \frac{0.61 \; x \; 450nm}{1.33 \; x \; 0.97}$$

$$d = 213 \text{ nm or } 0.213 \text{ μm}$$

Rubric 10: Industrial Hygiene Program Management

Corporations have resized and reorganized in recent years. This has led to fewer layers of management, fewer individual departments, and often the use of contract Health, Safety and Environmental professional services. Accordingly, it is important for the HSE professional to be proficient in business management, as well as technical industrial hygiene, safety and environmental practices.

Important Terms and Concepts

Accountability – The concept of being answerable for the end result. Accountability arises from responsibility.

Audit – A systematic review of a program or process. There are several types of audits, including: 1) Compliance audits, 2) Performance audits, and 3) System audits.

Delegation of Authority – A manager or team leader cannot perform all duties or direct all employees of a department and, therefore, assigns duties and responsibilities to subordinates. Typically, an effective span of control is 3-7 direct reports, with the ideal being 5.

Occupational Hygiene Audit – A multi-disciplinary, systematic process utilizing objective findings to evaluate the effectiveness of health and safety program components, as well as health and safety management systems. Historically, these were mainly compliance audits, but may be performance oriented. Audits should be performed by competent auditors. *Source: The Occupational Environment: Its Evaluation, Control and Management, 3rd edition*

Prevention through Design – Eliminating health and safety hazards during the design phase. This reduces the reliance on personal protective equipment and procedural controls. Installing equipment during the design phase is more successful and cost effective than implementing post design changes.

Risk Communication – The communication of risk to those affected or involved. It is typically two-way communication. To be effective, the communicator must be skilled in communication and credible regarding the content of the message. Some goals include: 1) Establishing or maintaining trust, 2) Involving effected persons, 3) Raising awareness, and 4) Improving decisions. *Source: The Occupational Environment: Its Evaluation, Control and Management, 3rd edition*

Risk Management – The identification, assessment, and prioritization of risks. ISO 31000 describes risk management as the effect of uncertainty upon objectives. It involves organized and economical use of resources to assess, reduce, and control the likelihood or magnitude of events. There are numerous risk management models with different goals and definitions depending on the context of application. Studies in Australia indicate that design is a significant contributor in 37% of work-related fatalities; therefore, the successful implementation of prevention through design concepts can have substantial impacts on worker health and safety.

ANSI/AIHA Z-10 – American National Standards Institute: Occupational Health and Safety Management System. It is characterized by continuous improvement and systematic elimination of the root causes of deficiencies.

ILO OHSMS – International Labor Office: Occupational Health and Safety Management System. It is an international management system focusing on integrated health and safety into business management and emphasizes that health and safety should be a line management function.

ISO 9001 – International Organization for Standardization: Quality Management System. It is an international consensus and certification process that focuses on continuous improvement in quality.

ISO 14001 – International Organization for Standardization: Environmental Management System. It is an international consensus and certification process that defines the elements of an effective environmental management.

OSHA Voluntary Protection Program – Occupational Safety and Health Administration (United States) voluntary safety management system.

OHSAS 18001- An international collaboration group and occupational health and safety consensus standard that has been adopted as a British standard.

Familiarity with both the content and intention of the American Board of Industrial Hygiene Code of Ethics is essential for the occupational hygiene professional.

Rubric 10: Industrial Hygiene Program Management Questions

1. Select the most important attribute of a successful Environmental, Health and Safety program.

    A) Sole responsibility of all program elements is assigned to the EHS manager.
    B) A high level of distribution of responsibilities for program actions among functional departments.
    C) The professional in charge has the word "manager" in his/her job title.
    D) The organizational culture must be defined in the written policy.

2. Select the answer that best describes the difference between strategic plan and operating plan.

    A) Integration of the industrial hygienist role is outlined in the strategic plan but not in the operating plan.
    B) Strategic planning is short term while operating plans span many years.
    C) The strategic plan describes the desired outcomes in a 3-5 year period while the operating plan establishes specific short term goals.
    D) Strategic plans are developed by the board of directors while the operational plan is developed at the operations level.

3. According to McGregor, Theory Y directs a people centered approach. Which of the following is not a basic assumption of theory Y?

    A) Work is not a normal part of life.
    B) People can exercise self-control and do not require threats to work effectively.
    C) People commit to objectives based on their perception of rewards.
    D) People seek responsibility.

4. Which of the following is not an AIHA Management System Component?

    A) Responsibility and authority.
    B) Inspection and evaluation.
    C) Define leadership.
    D) Communication systems.

5. Pliney the Elder (23-79 A.D.), a Roman Scholar, described the use of a crude respirator. What is the material of construction for this respirator?

    A) Sheep's wool.
    B) Tightly woven silk.
    C) Animal bladder.
    D) Crushed coal.

6. Who is credited with originating the statement, "All substances are poison; there is none that is not a poison. The dose separates the poison from the cure."

   A) Paracelcus.
   B) Bauer.
   C) Galen.
   D) Ellenbog.

7. When is it acceptable practice for a consulting industrial hygienist to provide sampling results directly to the worker who was evaluated?

   A) If the employee asks for the results.
   B) If the testing is being performed on Friday and the report must be sent before the end of the week.
   C) It is not acceptable to provide results directly to the worker.
   D) If the worker faces immediate serious hazard related to the exposure.

8. Select the best description of Participative Leadership.

   A) Direct people, explain decisions, react to change.
   B) Build trust, facilitate decisions, create a team identity.
   C) Involve people, develop individual performance, resolve conflicts.
   D) Contain conflict, get input, inspire teamwork.

9. Which of the following systems is designed to provide organizations with an effective tool for continual improvement of occupational health and safety performance?

   A) ISO 9001.
   B) ANSI/ASSE Z-10.
   C) ISO 14001.
   D) ANSI Z 87.1.

10. Select the best definition of a benchmark.

   A) A systematic means of ensuring that the demands of the customer are met.
   B) A formal process for performance data collection and analysis.
   C) A continuous improvement management system.
   D) A standard of performance against which similar processes can be measured.

11. Out of the following techniques listed below, which is most likely to result in a positive safety record at a company?

   A) Utilize and implement a safety tool that will evaluate facility safety.
   B) Conduct safety meetings only after major incidents have occurred.
   C) Fire the company safety director.
   D) Ensure supervisors and managers are accountable for safety.

12. Choose the statement that correctly identifies the key components of the Voluntary Protection Program.

    A) Management commitment and employee involvement, personal protective equipment, effective communication, and safety and health training.
    B) Management commitment and employee involvement, effective communication, hazard prevention and control, and safety and health training.
    C) Management commitment and employee involvement, worksite analysis, personal protective equipment, and safety and health training.
    D) Management commitment and employee involvement, worksite analysis, hazard prevention and control, and safety and health training.

13. Calculate the error of measurement if the true value is 20 ppm and the experimental value is 25 ppm.

    A) -20%
    B) -25%
    C) 20%
    D) 25%

14. According to a company's safety professional, the following estimated errors are present in a sampling system. Flow rate measurement $\pm 11\%$. Sampling time $\pm 2.8\%$. Collection efficiency $\pm 3.9\%$. Sample recovery $\pm 8.7\%$. Sample analysis $\pm 17\%$. Calculate the cumulative error for the sampling system.

    A) 10.1%
    B) 22.6%
    C) 34.5%
    D) 40.3%

15. Choose the answer that is a measure of reliability.

    A) Human and social factors.
    B) Physiological and psychological factors.
    C) Mean time to failure (MTF).
    D) Pre-time to post-time to failure.

16. Which of the following answers is not included in a Process Safety hazard analysis?

    A) Human factors.
    B) Quantitative proportion of employees and annual process injuries.
    C) Qualitative evaluation of failure of controls on employees.
    D) Facility siting.

17. An IH takes numerous samples at an operation. The IH notices there is a lot of variability among the analysis. The analysis displays a few high samples relative to the rest. The term that describes this variability is?

    A) Log-normal distribution.
    B) Normal distribution.
    C) Poisson Distribution.
    D) Gaussian Distribution.

18. Select the statement that best describes the concepts of Taguchi Experiments.

    A) Obtaining and considering the opinion of experts.
    B) Listing criteria under two headings to overcome personal preference.
    C) Comparison of existing programs to world class programs.
    D) A method for evaluating several elements of a process at the same time.

19. According to Maslow's theory on the hierarchy of needs, which condition must be satisfied before any other need can be addressed?

    A) Safety and security.
    B) Physiological.
    C) Self-esteem.
    D) Self-fulfillment.

20. The following 7 components are sequential steps in which management approach? Identification of key business objectives and hazards; conduct risk assessments; align value opportunities; identify impacts; measure impacts; determine value; and value presentation.

    A) The AIHA Value Strategy.
    B) ANSI Z-10 Value sub-section B.
    C) The 7 Values of Successful Operations.
    D) ISO Risk Management.

Rubric 10: Industrial Hygiene Program Management Answers

1. **Answer B.**
   Explanation: Every organization should have a clearly stated policy that articulates the company's commitment to EHS and distributes responsibilities to functional departments or groups within the organization. If the departments understand and accept their responsibilities, then the EHS values will likely become part of the company culture.
   Source: The Occupational Environment: It's Evaluation, Control, and Management, 3rd Edition

2. **Answer C.**
   Explanation: Strategic plans focus on long term issues and may change periodically with changes in business. Operating plans are typically fixed goals for one or two year time periods. High profile EHS activities should be included in the operating plan, and ongoing EHS issues should be included in the strategic plan.
   Source: The Occupational Environment: It's Evaluation, Control, and Management, 3rd Edition

3. **Answer A.**
   Explanation: Theory Y states people view work as normal and do not dislike it, and most people can be innovative and tend to use a small portion of their intellectual potential. Theory Y workplaces tend to be participative in nature.
   Source: The Occupational Environment: It's Evaluation, Control, and Management, 3rd Edition

4. **Answer C.**
   Explanation: According to the AIHA Management Systems Criteria, the answer selection "Define leadership" is not an AIHA Management System Component. Responsibility and authority warrants that all members of an organization are accountable for safety and health issues, and members know their roles and responsibilities. Inspection and evaluation determines a protocol to regularly inspect and audit the workplace for safety and health defects. Communication systems develop and implement procedures to express safety and health requirements to employees and contractors to prevent or mitigate potential exposures and hazards. The other AIHA Management System Criteria include health and safety policy; resources; written documentation; procedures; planning; compliance and conformance review; goals and objectives; design control; document and data control; purchasing; corrective and preventive action; and training.

5. **Answer C.**
   Explanation: Animal bladders were used at this time to prevent the inhalation of 'pernicious dust' associated with mining.
   Source: Applications and Computational Elements of Industrial Hygiene, Stern and Mansdorf

6. **Answer A.**
   Explanation: Paracelcus was a Swiss physician and proponent of observational medicine. His statement has become a foundation for toxicology and dose response. Bauer published a 12 volume work titled *De Re Metallica*. Bauer's Latin name is Georgius Agricola.
   Source: Applications and Computational Elements of Industrial Hygiene, Stern and Mansdorf

7. Answer D.

   Explanation: According the American Board of Industrial Hygiene Code of Ethics, a CIH or candidate has a responsibility to maintain and respect the confidentiality of sensitive information obtained in the course of professional activities, unless:
   - The information is reasonably understood to pertain to unlawful activity
   - A court or governmental agency lawfully directs the release of the information
   - The client or employer expressly authorizes the release of specific information
   - The failure to release such information would likely result in death or serious physical harm to the employee or the public

8. Answer C.

   Explanation:

   <u>Supervisory leadership</u> includes directing people, explaining decisions, reacting to change, and containing conflict.

   <u>Team leadership</u> includes building trust, facilitating decisions, creating a team identity, foreseeing and influencing change, building trust, and inspiring teamwork.

   <u>Participative Leadership</u> includes involving people, developing individual performance, resolving conflicts, receiving input, and developing individual performance.

   Source: The Occupational Environment: It's Evaluation, Control, and Management, 3rd Edition

9. Answer B.

   Explanation: ISO 9001 is a Quality Management System, ISO 14001 is an Environmental Management System, ISO 19011 is Quality and Environmental Management Auditing, ANSI Z 87.1 addresses eye and face protection.

10. Answer D.

    Explanation: Benchmarks allow for comparing a program to other well-regarded programs to determine areas of potential improvement. The process is most effective when carried out by the employees who are responsible for the benchmarked activity.

    Source: The Occupational Environment: It's Evaluation, Control, and Management, 3rd Edition

11. Answer D.

    Explanation: The greatest impact on safety at any company is line management. In order to ensure a positive safety record, line management should be held accountable for their safety performance.

12. Answer D.

    Explanation: The key components to OSHA's Voluntary Protection Program include management commitment and employee involvement; worksite analysis; hazard prevention and control; and safety and health training.

    Source: www.osha.gov

13. Answer D.
   Explanation:
   Step 1: Solve for percent error

$$\% \ error = \frac{(EV - TV)}{TV}$$

$$EV = 25 \ ppm$$
$$TV = 20 \ ppm$$

$$\% \ error = \frac{(25 \ ppm - 20 \ ppm)}{20 \ ppm}$$

$$\% \ error = 0.25 \ x \ 100$$

$$\% \ error = 25\%$$

14. Answer B.
   Explanation:
   Step 1: Solve for the cumulative error

$$E_c = \sqrt{[(E_1)^2 + (E_2)^2 + (E_3)^2 + (E_4)^2 + (E_5)^2]}$$

$$E_c = sampling \ system \ cumulative \ error \ (\%)$$
$$E_i = error \ number \ i \ (\%)$$

$$E_1 = 11\%$$
$$E_2 = 2.8\%$$
$$E_3 = 3.9\%$$
$$E_4 = 8.7\%$$
$$E_5 = 17\%$$

$$E_c = \sqrt{[(11)^2 + (2.8)^2 + (3.9)^2 + (8.7)^2 + (17)^2]}$$

$$E_c = \sqrt{121 + 7.8 + 15.2 + 75.7 + 289}$$

$$E_c = \sqrt{508.7}$$

$$E_c = 22.6\%$$

15. Answer C.

    Explanation: A term for measuring system reliability is probability of successful performance. Another measure of reliability is mean time to failure (MTF). MTF is defined as the amount of time that a system or individual performs successfully until a failure or between failures. Reliability engineering relates closely to safety engineering and to system safety; they use common methods for their analysis and may require input from each other. Reliability engineering focuses on costs of failure caused by system downtime, cost of spares, repair equipment, personnel, and cost of warranty claims. Safety engineering normally emphasizes not cost, but preserving life and nature, and therefore deals only with particular dangerous system-failure modes. High reliability levels also result from good engineering and from attention to detail, and almost never from only reactive failure management.
    Source: Barnard, R.W.A. (2008). What is wrong with Reliability Engineering

16. Answer B.

    Explanation: The following are parts involved in a process safety hazard analysis: facility siting, human factors, and qualitative evaluation of failure of controls on employees.
    Source: www.osha.gov

17. Answer A.

    Explanation: Sampling data usually follow a log-normal distribution. A normal distribution describes population data.
    Source: The Occupational Environment: Its Evaluation, Control and Management, 3rd. Edition

18. Answer D.

    Explanation: Decision making tools include the following:
    - Considered opinion - Obtaining and considering the opinion of experts
    - Factor Analysis Matrix - Listing criteria under two headings to overcome personal preference
    - Benchmarking - Comparison of existing programs to world class programs
    - Taguchi Experiments - A method for evaluating several elements of a process at the same time.
    Source: Industrial Hygiene Reference and Study Guide, 3rd Edition

19. Answer B.

    Explanation: Physiological needs include food, water, and shelter, which must be met before any other need.
    Source: Industrial Hygiene Reference and Study Guide, 3rd Edition

20. Answer A.

    Explanation: These are the components of the AIHA Value Strategy Model.
    Source: Industrial Hygiene Reference and Study Guide, 3rd Edition

Rubric 11: Noise

According to NIOSH, four million workers are exposed to high levels of noise, ten million people in the U.S. have a noise-related hearing loss, and twenty-two million workers are exposed to potentially damaging noise each year. Noise exposure can contribute to hearing loss, miscommunication, and emotional stress. The first sustained effort in hearing conservation was documented by the United States Military from soldiers returning home from World War II with noticeable hearing loss. The first documented enforcement of noise in the workplace came as part of the 1971 Noise Standard by OSHA.

Important Terms and Concepts

Audible Range – The frequency range across which normal ears hear is approximately 20 HZ to 20,000 HZ in undamaged ears.

Audiogram – A record of hearing loss or hearing level measured at several different frequencies – usually 500 Hz – 6,000 Hz.

Decibel – A unit to express sound-power level (Lw) and sound pressure level (Lp). Sound power is the total acoustic output of a source in watts (W). By definition, sound power level, in decibels, is Lw= 10 Log W/Wo, where W= sound power of the source and Wo is the reference sound power level of 10^{-12}. Because the decibel is also used to describe other physical quantities such as electric current and electrical voltage, the correct reference quantity must be specified.

dBA – Sound level in decibels read on the A scale of a sound-level meter. The A scale discriminates against very low frequencies (as does the human ear) and is, therefore, better for measuring general sound levels.

dBC – Sound level in decibels read on the C scale of a sound-level meter. The C scale discriminates very little against low frequencies.

Hertz (HZ) – The frequency measured in cycles per second, 1 cps = 1Hz.

Noise – Any unwanted sound.

Continuous Noise – A broadband of noise of approximately constant level and spectrum for an extended period of time.

Impact Noise – A sharp burst of noise.

Intermittent noise – A broadband of noise that is experienced several times for shorter durations.

Noise Reduction – Sound pressure level difference between two spaces separated by a barrier.

Noise Reduction Rating (NRR) – A rating developed by the Environmental Protection Agency (EPA) that allows for determining the adequacy of hearing protection for a given sound pressure level.

Octave Band – A range of frequencies where the upper band of the upper band-edge frequency is double the lower band frequency. Knowing the frequency and band allows for more effective control measures.

Sound Pressure Level (SPL) – The level, in decibels, of a sound is 20 times the $\log_{10}$ of the ratio of the pressure of this sound to the reference pressure, which must be explicitly stated.

Standard Threshold Shift – An average loss of hearing acuity in either ear of 10 dB as averaged over the 2,000, 3,000 and 4,000-hertz frequencies.

Temporary Threshold Shift (TTS) – The hearing loss suffered as the result of noise exposure, all or part of which is recovered during an arbitrary period of time when one is removed from the noise. It accounts for the necessity of checking hearing acuity at least 16 hours after a noise exposure.

Physics of Sound

Sound Power

$$L_W = 10 \, log \, \frac{W}{W_0}$$

Where:

L_W is the sound power level expressed as dB

W is the power expressed in Watts

W_0 is the reference power, a constant of 10^{-12} Watts

Use: To determine the sound power level in dB without taking into account the configuration of the space. Measuring sound power level is very difficult, which is why the sound pressure level formula is used as the preferred alternative.

Example:

Your home is located next to a highway that has a sound power of approximately 0.01 Watts. What would the Sound Power Level be in dB?

$$L_W = 10 \, log \, \frac{W}{W_0}$$

Step 1: Solve for L_W

$$L_W = 10 \, log \, \frac{0.01 \; watts}{10^{-12} \; watts}$$

$$L_W = 100 \, dB$$

Sound Pressure

$$SPL \ or \ L_p = 20 \ log\left(\frac{P}{P_0}\right)$$

Where:
SPL is the sound pressure level, expressed as dB
SPL may be L_p in equations
P is the measured root mean squared sound pressure, expressed as Pa
P_0 is the reference root mean squared sound pressure, expressed as Pa
(0.00002 Pa or 20 uPa)

Use: To determine the sound pressure level radiated by a source when the sound pressure level in Pa or uPa is known.

Example:
Calculate the sound pressure level in dB when the measured root mean squared sound pressure is 0.4 Pa?

$$SPL = 20log\left(\frac{P}{P_0}\right)$$

Step 1: Solve for SPL

$$SPL = 20log\left(\frac{0.4 \ Pa}{0.00002 \ Pa}\right)$$

$$SPL = 86 \ dB$$

Sound Pressure Level from Identical Sources

$$SPL_f = SPL_i + 10 \log(n)$$

Where:

SPL_f is the total sound pressure obtained by combining n identical sources, expressed as (dB)

SPL_i is the sound pressure level of each source, expressed as (dB)

n is the total number of sources.

Use:

To determine the potential sound pressure level during the design phase or for identifying areas that may require hearing protection.

Note: This formula requires that all noise sources are the same sound pressure level in a free field.

Useful Approximation

Numerical differences between sound pressure levels	*Amount added to the higher sound pressure level*
0-1	3
2-4	2
5-9	1
>10	0

Example:

A company produces parts that require industrial fans to cool the finished product in an open space. Currently the operation has one industrial fan that operates at a sound pressure level (SPL) of 86 dB. Due to production increases, The ompany has purchased three additional industrial fans for the area. What would the expected SPL be in the area once they are installed?

$$SPL_f = SPL_i + 10 \log(n)$$

Step 1: Solve for SPL_f

$$SPL_f = 86 + 10 \log(4)$$

$$SPL_f = 92 \text{ dB}$$

Rule of Thumb

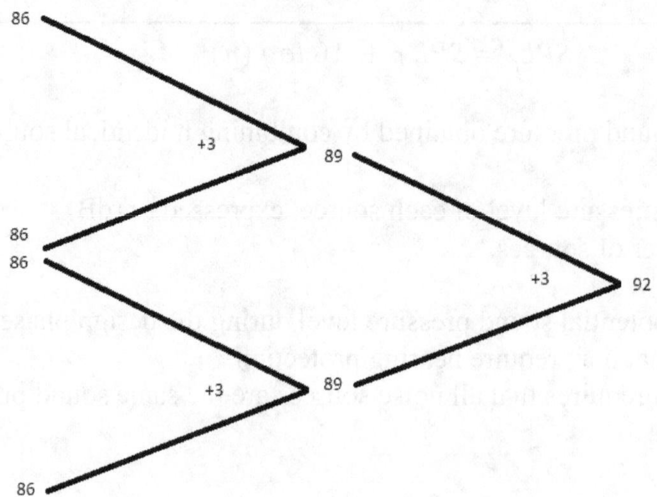

Adding Sound Pressure Level from Different Sources

$$L_{PT} = 10 \, log \sum 10^{\frac{L_i}{10}}$$

Where:

$L \; or \; SPL_f$ is the resulting sound pressure level obtained by summing levels of each sound pressure level (L or SPL), expressed as dB.

$L_i \; or \; SPL_i$ is the sound pressure levels from each individual source.

Use: To determine the potential sound pressure level during the design phase or for identifying areas that may require hearing protection.

Note: This formula can be used for identical sources or non-identical sound sources.

Rule of thumb method

Numerical differences between sound pressure levels	*Amount added to the higher sound pressure level*
0-1	3
2-4	2
5-9	1
>10	0

Example:

As part of an ongoing expansion project, your company is planning on adding two additional high efficiency exhaust fans to a chemical room. The literature on the fans states that each individual fan operates at 85 dB. The room already has three fans that operate at 89 dB individually. What would the expected noise level be after the new fans are installed?

$$L_{PT} = 10 \, log \sum 10^{\frac{L_i}{10}}$$

Step 1: Solve for L_{PT}

$$SPL_f = 10 \, log \left(10^{\frac{85}{10}} + 10^{\frac{85}{10}} + 10^{\frac{89}{10}} + 10^{\frac{89}{10}} + 10^{\frac{89}{10}}\right)$$

$$L_{PT} = 94.7 \, dB$$

Example 2:
Three machines are going to be situated in close proximity. Given their individual sound pressure levels, L_{Pi}, of 80, 84 and 87 dB. What is the approximate total sound pressure level?

$$L_{PT} = 10 \, log \left(\sum_{i=1}^{N} 10^{\frac{L_{Pi}}{10}} \right)$$

Step 1: Solve for L_{PT}

$$L_{PT} = 10 \, log \left(10^{\frac{80}{10}} + 10^{\frac{84}{10}} + 10^{\frac{87}{10}} \right)$$

$$L_{PT} = 89 \, dB$$

Average Sound Pressure Level

$$L_{eq} = 10\,log\left[\frac{1}{T}\sum_{i=1}^{N}\left(10^{\frac{L_i}{10}}xt_i\right)\right]$$

Where:
L_{eq} is equivalent (or average) sound pressure level in dB
L_i is the sound pressure level dB for i period of time
T is the total time of the observation period
t_i is the interval of time for which a sound pressure level is obtained
N is the number of time increments
T is the total time
Rewritten:

$$L_{eq} = 10\,log\left(\frac{\left(10^{\frac{L_1}{10}} x\, t_1\right) + \left(10^{\frac{L_2}{10}} x\, t_2\right) \dots}{T}\right)$$

Example: A gas turbine operates on a cyclical basis. The turbine owners must build a wall if the average sound pressure exceeds 80 dB over a 24-hour period. Field evaluation with an SLM yield the following: 3 periods of 90 dB each lasting 4 hours, 1 period of 70 dB for 8-hours, 1 period of 80 dB for 4-hours. What is the average and should a wall be constructed?

$$L_{eq} = 10\,log\left(\frac{\left(10^{\frac{90}{10}} x\, 12\right) + \left(10^{\frac{70}{10}} x\, 8\right) + \left(10^{\frac{80}{10}} x\, 4\right)}{24}\right)$$

L_{eq} = 87 dB, so yes build a wall

Sound Pressure Level and Distance

$$SPL_2 = SPL_1 + 20\ log\left(\frac{d_1}{d_2}\right)$$

Where:
SPL_2 is the sound pressure level for distance d_2 expressed as dB
SPL_1 is the sound pressure level for distance d_1 expressed as dB
d_1 is the initial distance (keep distance units the same as d_2)
d_2 is the second distance (keep distance units the same as d_1)

Use: Determining the potential sound pressure levels at a given distance when the sound pressure level is known at another distance.

Note: In a free field as sound travels further from the source, the sound pressure level decreases in a ratio proportional to the square of the distance.

The 6 dB rule states that if distance from the noise source is doubled, subtract 6 dB. If the distance is reduced by 1/2, then add 6 dB.

Example:
A single air compressor is located in the middle of a room segregated from all other operations. The air compressor operates at a noise level of 98 dB at 5 feet. What would the noise level be at 12 feet?

$$SPL_2 = SPL_1 + 20\ log\left(\frac{d_1}{d_2}\right)$$

Step 1: Solve for SPL_2

$$SPL_2 = 96 + 20\ log\left(\frac{5}{12}\right)$$

$$SPL_2 = 88.4\ dB$$

Maximum Exposure Time

$$T = \frac{8}{2^{\left(SPL-90/5\right)}}$$

Where:

T is the maximum amount of time that a worker can be exposed to a given sound pressure level without anticipated adverse outcomes

SPL is the sound pressure level, expressed as (dB)

Use: The time a worker can be exposed to a constant sound pressure level without adverse effects or compliance issues.

Note: The average sound pressure level for a shift can be used to calculate the dose % for that shift.

Alternate:

$$T_p = \frac{T_c}{2^{\left(L_{AS}-\frac{L_C}{ER}\right)}}$$

Where:

T_P is the maximum amount of time that a worker can be exposed to a given sound pressure level without anticipated adverse effects

T_c is the time allowed based on the criterion level L_C

L_{AS} is the sound level measured on the A scale, slow response

L_C is the criterion level (100% of dose- OSHA 90 dBA and ACGIH 85 dBA)

ER is the exchange rate (OSHA 5 and ACGIH 3)

Example:

Bag handlers at the airport are exposed to 112 dB while unloading bags. Assuming no controls are available to control the noise, how long can they work in that environment without assumed adverse effects?

$$T = \frac{8}{2^{\left(SPL-90/5\right)}}$$

Step 1: Solve for T

$$T = \frac{8}{2^{\left(112-90/5\right)}}$$

$$T = \frac{8}{21.1}$$

$$T = 0.379 \; Hours = 23 \; minutes$$

Allowed Noise Exposure Time - ACGIH

$$Time = \frac{8}{2^{\left(\frac{L-85}{3}\right)}}$$

Where:
T is the allowed exposure time expressed in hours
L is the sound pressure level expressed in dBA

Use: To calculate the allowed exposure times during a 10-hour work day following the ACGIH TLV standard.

Example:
A company has employees who work 10-hour shifts. What is the ACGIH noise exposure limit for the 10-hour shift?

$$Time = \frac{8}{2^{\left(\frac{L-85}{3}\right)}}$$

Step 1: Rearrange the equation

$$10 = \frac{8}{2^{\left(\frac{L-85}{3}\right)}}$$

$$2^{\left(\frac{L-85}{3}\right)} = \frac{8}{10}$$

$$log2\left(\frac{L-85}{3}\right) = log\left(\frac{8}{10}\right)$$

$$\left(\frac{L-85}{3}\right)0.30103 = 0.09691$$

Step 2: Solve for L

$$L = 3\left(\frac{-0.09691}{0.30103}\right) + 85 = 84.0\ dBA$$

Percentage Dose Based Upon Exposure Time

$$\%D = 100\left(\frac{C_1}{T_1} + \frac{C_2}{T_2} + \cdots + \frac{C_i}{T_i}\right)$$

Where:

$\%D$ is the percentage of allowable noise dose. Anything over 100% would indicate an overexposure to noise.

C_1 is the duration of exposure for T_1, expressed as hours

C_i is the duration of exposure for T_i, expressed as hours

$T_1 \ldots T_i$ are the corresponding amount of times permitted at a certain exposure level, expressed as hours. T can be calculated or can be derived from OSHA table G-16.

Use: To determine noise dose percentage for a worker when personal noise dosimetry cannot be used. The dose can be used to determine the workers TWA.

Allowable Noise Exposure

OSHA 5 decibel (dBb) Exchange	ACGIH 3 decibel (db) Exchange
105 db → 1 hour	94 db → 1 hour
100 db → 2 hours	91 db → 2 hours
95 db → 4 hours	88 db → 4 hours
90 db → 8 hours	85 db → 8 hours
85 db → 16 hours	82 db → 16 hours

Note: Neither incorporate sounds levels under 80 db into dose.

Example:

During the course of an 8-hour work day, one employee was exposed to the following noise levels: 97 dBA for 3 hours, 90 dBA for 3 hours, and 92 dBA for 2 hours. What is the employee's percent dose exposure?

$$\%D = 100\left(\frac{C_1}{T_1} + \frac{C_2}{T_2} + \frac{C_3}{T_3}\right)$$

Step 1: Solve for Dose %

$$\%D = 100\left(\frac{3}{3} + \frac{3}{8} + \frac{2}{6}\right)$$

$$\%D = 171$$

Time Weighted Average Based Upon Dose Percentage

$$TWA = 16.61 \, log \left(\frac{\%D}{100}\right) + 90 \, dBA$$

Where:

TWA is the time weighted average, expressed in dBA

$\%D$ is the dose of the exposure, this can be measured or calculated

Use: To express total dose observed or calculated as a TWA for compliance or control measure selection.

Example:

Given a dose of 171%, determine what the Time Weighted Average would be.

$$TWA = 16.61 \, log \left(\frac{\%D}{100}\right) + 90 \, dBA$$

Step 1: Solve for TWA

$$TWA = 16.61 \, Log_{10} \, \frac{171}{100} + 90$$

$$TWA = 3.87 + 90$$

$$TWA = 93.8$$

TWA$_{eq}$ Calculated from % Dose (TLV)

$$TWA_{eq} = 10\ log\left(\frac{\%D}{100}\right) + 85 dBA$$

Where:

TWA$_{eq}$ is the equivalent time weighted average exposure, expressed as dBA
%D is the dose of the exposure, this can be measured or calculated

Use: To calculate the dose and TWA to the ACGIH TLV of 85 dBA and incorporates 3 dB exchange rate.

Example:
A worker is monitored for noise exposure, and the dosimeter readout indicated a dose of 320%. Using the ACHIH criteria, what is the TWA$_{eq}$ exposure in dBA?

$$TWA_{eq} = 10\ log\left(\frac{\%D}{100}\right) + 85 dBA$$

Step 1: Solve for TWA$_{eq}$

$$TWA_{eq} = 10\ log\left(\frac{\%D}{100}\right) + 85 dBA$$

$$TWA_{eq} = 10\ log\left(\frac{320}{100}\right) + 85$$

$$TWA_{eq} = 10\ log(3.2) + 85$$

$$TWA_{eq} = 10\ (0.505) + 85$$

$$TWA_{eq} = 90\ dBA$$

Evaluating Sound

Dosimetry

Noise dosimeters are the primary method for measuring worker noise exposure. There are three primary methods that noise is measured using the dosimeter:

OSHA Hearing Conservation Program – Used primarily to determine whether or not employees need to be placed in a company sponsored hearing conservation program according to OSHA 1910.95 (c) 1. The settings are:
- Range: 80-130 dB
- Exchange rate: 5 dB
- Frequency rating: A Scale
- Response: Slow
- TWA: 85 dB
- Dose Threshold: 50%

OSHA Compliance – Used by OSHA to determine compliance to the 1910.95 standard.
- Range: 90-115 dB
- Exchange rate: 5 dB
- Frequency rating: A Scale
- Response: Slow
- TWA 90 dB – aka criterion
- Dose Threshold: 100%

ACGIH – Not Compliance
- Range: 80-140 dB
- Exchange rate: 3 dB
- Frequency rating: A Scale
- Response: Slow
- TWA 85 dB – aka criterion
- Dose Threshold: 100%

The dosimeter serves two functions when used: 1) Captures sound pressure levels in the hearing zone of the employee, and 2) Computes the data based upon the chosen settings.

Sound Level Meters

Sound level meters (SLM) are portable devices use for obtaining noise measurements. The primary use of SLMs is to take spot measurements of noise levels, which can assist in determining when and where controls are best suited. Depending on the application of the SLM, there are *four types* that can be used.

> **Type 0** – Laboratory standard: used in a laboratory as a reference standard
> **Type 1** – Precision: can be used in the laboratory or field with an error level not exceeding 1 dB
> **Type 2** – General purpose: intended for general field use with an error level not exceeding 2 dB
> **Type S** – May have design tolerances of any of the three grades, but it is not required to contain all functions of a non-special purpose sound level meter

Sound Level Surveys

Sound level surveys are conducted in the field to determine which areas of a facility or worksite need additional noise evaluation. The sound level survey is used to develop a baseline noise exposure, which can be used to determine the need for personal dosimetry. According to OSHA, anytime noise levels of 80 dB or higher are found during a sound level survey, additional noise sampling should be conducted.

Frequency analyzers

Frequency analyzers are used by the industrial hygienist to determine sound pressure levels across one or more bandwidths. The main frequency analyzer used in the field for noise measurements is the Octave Band analyzer. Depending on the octave band analyzer used, it may read in octaves or 1/3 octaves. Octave band analyzers that take readings in 1/3 octaves are more specific than whole octave measurements. Frequency analyzers are very closely related to SLM's with the most important difference being that the analyzers can determine the difference of sound pressure levels at different octaves. Octave bands are based upon the center frequency of the upper and lower sound bands. The following table shows the center frequencies, and the upper and lower bands used in octave band (1/1) analysis.

Table: Frequencies of 1/1 Octave Bands

Lower Bandwidth (Hz)	Center Frequency	Upper bandwidth (Hz)
22	31.5	44
44	63	88
88	125	177
177	250	354
354	500	707
707	1000	1414
1414	2000	2828
2828	4000	5656
5656	8000	11312
11312	16000	22624

The relationship between the weighting scales is shown in the table below:

Sound Level Meter Scales

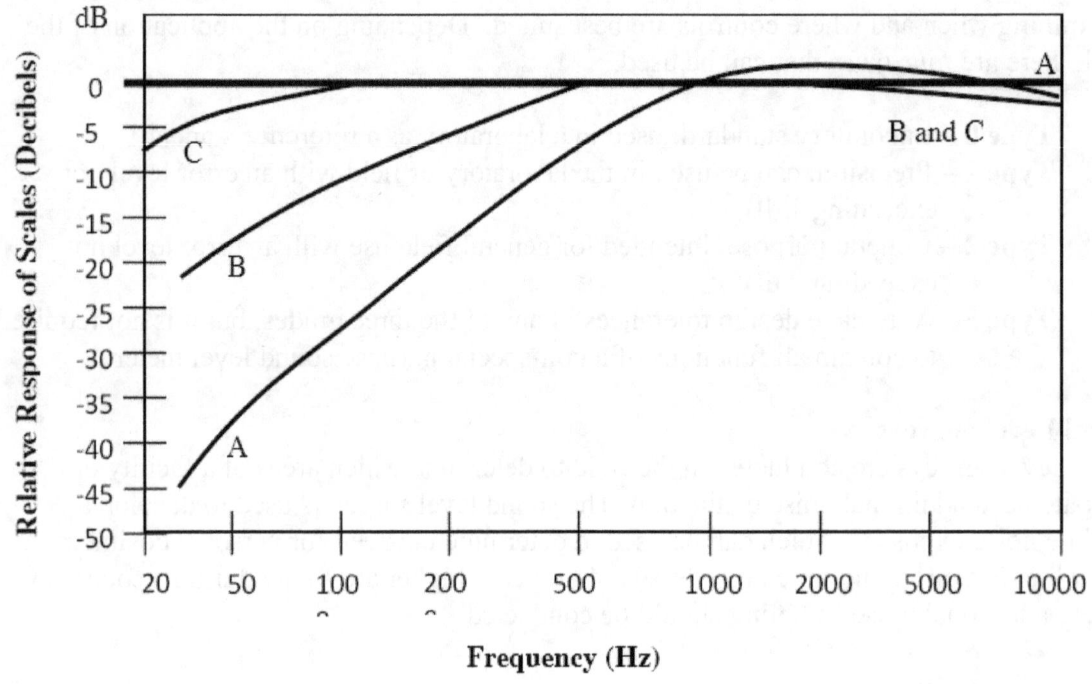

SPAN Image

Sound Fields

<u>**Sound field**</u> – A region in which sound is propagating.

- *Free Field* – A region in which there are no reflected sound waves. In a free field, sound radiates in all directions uniformly.

- *Near Field* – The area within one wavelength of the noise source. Noise measurements within the near field are generally not accurate because small changes in microphone position can have big effects on noise readings.

- *Far Field* – The area that is greater than one wavelength from the noise source. Noise measurements in the far field are generally accurate but if the noise source is not located in a free field, the noise readings can be effected by the reverberant field.

- *Reverberant Field* – The area where the reflected sound dominates the noise source.

Sound fields exist wherever there is a noise source. Within a diffuse sound field, the sound pressure level is reduced by 6 dB when the distance is doubled. However, within the work place a diffuse sound field is seldom encountered, thus making it difficult to estimate sound pressure levels coming directly from the sound source.

Noise Reduction by Source Treatment

Source treatment involves stopping the sound before it can reach the employees in the work area. There are four ways to treat the noise at source.

1) **Modification** – Equipment that has mechanical parts, high pressure flows or vibrating parts can cause high noise levels in the workplace. An effective way to manage noise levels from mechanical parts is to maintain the equipment up to the manufacturer's specifications and have a well-developed preventative maintenance plan. This will ensure no excess noise is generated from the source.

2) **Retrofit** – Retrofitting a noise source involves installing a product designed to reduce noise at the source. These products are designed to be used in close proximity to the source to prevent transmission of sound. Examples include:

   - *Vibration damping materials*- Typically installed at the noise source to reduce the amount of vibration generated, which reduces noise levels.

   - *Vibration isolating devices* – Vibration isolating devices can be installed to assist in noise control by limiting the amount of vibration transmitted through solid surfaces. Examples of applications of vibration isolating devices are:

     - Using pipe hangers on high velocity pipes that tend to vibrate
     - Using flexible connections in piping and ductwork
     - Installing rotating mounts on equipment to reduce vibration

   - *Silencers* – Silencers are inserted into a flowing medium, typically air, to reduce the noise level downstream. Sound absorbing materials are used in areas with high levels of reverberant noise. As hard surfaces around the noise source reflect the sound, it can build up, thus causing the sound pressure level in the area to increase. A disadvantage of installing sound absorptive material is that it does not address the noise coming from the noise source.

3) **Substitution** – Substitution of a piece of equipment with a lower noise level piece is a viable noise control method. Examples of this include:

   - Installing belts to replace gears
   - Installing conveyors to replace rollers
   - Replacing metal components with components with high internal dampening components, such as rubber or plastic
   - Using perforated or mesh components in place of solid metal to reduce vibration

 Copyright©2019 SPAN International Training, LLC

4) **Relocation** – In some applications, a noise source can be moved or transferred to areas where it poses less of a hazard to employees. Examples of relocating the noise source include the following:

- Moving pneumatic components to eliminate noise exposure from air discharge ports and pneumatic exhausts
- Routing high flow hydraulic pipes, pumps and blowers to a non-occupied area

Noise Reduction by Path Treatment

When it is not possible to reduce sound at the source, the next viable option is to treat the noise at the transmission path. Treating the sound during transmission can be done in many ways, but the three most prominent ways are by adding sound absorption material, installing acoustical enclosures and adding acoustical barriers. The most common engineering control for path treatment of sound is acoustical enclosures.

Acoustical Enclosures

The two primary methods that are used to determine the effectiveness of a noise enclosure are **transmission loss** and **insertion loss**. Transmission loss is the reduction of sound pressure level due to the insertion of a partition, barrier, or enclosure. Insertion loss is the difference of sound pressure levels at a fixed measurement location as taken before and after inserting a noise enclosure.

Transmission loss refers to the coefficient of transmission for the material that the enclosure is constructed from while the insertion loss refers to the effectiveness of the enclosure at a location before and after installation. The maximum insertion loss that can be achieved is the transmission loss for the material the enclosure is constructed from.

In order to calculate transmission loss, the transmission coefficient (τ) must be known. The following table has a list of general construction materials and their transmission coefficient.

Table: Approximate Transmission Loss for Materials (dB)

Material	125	250	500	1,000	2,000	4,000
				Hz		
Sheet metal laminate, 2 lb/ft^2, viscoelastic core	15	25	28	32	39	42
Steel, 16 gauge, 2.5 lb/ft^2	21	30	34	37	40	47
Steel, 18 gauge, 2 lb/ft^2	15	19	31	32	35	48
Plywood, ¾ inch, 2 lb/ft^2	24	22	27	28	25	27
Plywood, ¼ inch, 0.7 lb/ft^2	17	15	20	24	28	27
Panels, perforated metal with mineral fiber tile, 4 inch thick	28	34	40	48	56	62
Glass, laminated, ½ inch	23	31	38	40	47	52
Glass, plate. ¼ inch	25	29	33	36	26	35
Fiber tile, filled mineral, $\frac{5}{8}$ inch	30	32	39	43	53	60
Door, hardwood, 2 $\frac{5}{8}$ inch	26	33	40	43	48	51
Curtains, lead vinyl, 1 ½ lb/ft^2	22	23	25	31	35	42
Concrete block, 6 inch, lightweight, painted	38	36	40	45	50	56
Cinder block, 7 $\frac{5}{8}$ inch, hollow	33	33	33	39	45	51
Brick, 4 inch	30	36	37	37	37	43

Transmission Loss

$$TL = 10 \, log\left(\frac{E_i}{E_t}\right)$$

$$TL = 10 \, log\left(\frac{1}{\tau}\right), dB$$

There are 2 transmission loss formulas in noise references. The second formula is considered a simpler form and is shown on 2017 ABIH formula sheet.

Where:
TL is the reduction of sound pressure level due to the insertion of a partition, barrier, or enclosure
τ is the ratio of sound energy transmitted through a wall unit area to the sound energy on the wall

Use: To determine the sound pressure reduction at a fixed measurement location with the installation of a noise enclosure.

Example:
If a noise enclosure is constructed ¼" plywood, calculate the expected transmission loss at 1000 Hz.

$$TL = 10 \, log\left(\frac{1}{\tau}\right)$$

Step 1: Locate the τ value for ¼ inch plywood at 1000 Hz on the transmission loss table: 24

Step 2: Solve for TL

$$TL = 10 \, log\left(\frac{1}{24}\right)$$

$$TL = -14 \, dB$$

Source: The Noise Manual 5th ed. AIHA

Insertion Loss

Insertion loss refers to the amount of sound reduction achieved by installing a noise enclosure. Generally, the greater the amount of insertion loss the more effective the noise enclosure.

Insertion Loss

$$IL = SPL_{Out1} - SPL_{Out2}, dB$$

Where:

IL is the difference of sound pressure levels at a fixed measurement location, taken prior to and after inserting a noise enclosure

SPL_{Out1} is the sound pressure level outside the enclosure prior to installation of the enclosure

SPL_{Out2} is the sound pressure level outside the enclosure after the installation of the enclosure

Use: To determine the sound pressure reduction at a fixed measurement location with the installation of a noise enclosure

Note: Not on 2017 ABIH formula sheet

Example:

Measured at 5-feet from the noise source, the reading is 96 dB. After a noise enclosure was installed, measurements were repeated at 5-feet from the noise source and sound pressure level was 88 dB. Calculate insertion loss of the noise enclosure.

$$IL = SPL_{Out1} - SPL_{Out2}$$

Step 1: Solve for IL

$$IL = 96 - 88$$

$$IL = 8\ dB$$

Source: The Noise Manual, 5th Edition AIHA

Personal Protective Equipment

When suitable engineering controls cannot be established, the final way to control noise control is Personal Protective Equipment (PPE). PPE for noise controls are generally referred to as Hearing Protection Devices (HPD).

Inserts – Can be made from several different materials and they are designed to be inserted into the ear canal to reduce noise exposure.

Earmuffs – Consist of a hard shell outside and a cushion that fits tightly around the outside of the ear.

$$Estimated\ Noise\ Exposure = TWA - \left(\frac{NRR - 7}{2}\right)$$

Where:
Estimated Noise Exposure is the sound pressure level, expressed as dBA
TWA is the sound pressure level to which an employee is exposed, expressed as dBA
NRR is the noise reduction rating listed on the hearing protection device

Use: To estimate the sound pressure level an employee is exposed to when wearing a specific type of hearing protection device.

Note: Subtract seven from the NRR if the TWA is measured in dBA. If the TWA is measured in dBC, do not subtract seven. The result of the NRR-7 is divided by 2 to take into account derating of the hearing protection. The NRR is not divided by 2 for OSHA compliance purposes.

Note: Not on the 2017 ABIH formula sheet.

Example:
Based upon industrial hygiene sampling conducted in and around a steel mill, an employee has an 8-hour TWA of 96 decibels. The hearing protection inserts the employee is using have an NRR of 29 dB. Considering the employee has been trained and is using the inserts correctly, what is the estimated noise exposure for the employee?

$$Estimated\ Noise\ Exposure = TWA - \left(\frac{NRR - 7}{2}\right)$$

Step 1: Solve for Estimated Noise Exposure

$$Estimated\ Noise\ Exposure = 96 - \left(\frac{29 - 7}{2}\right)$$

$$Estimated\ Noise\ Exposure = 96 - 11$$

$$Estimated\ Noise\ Exposure = 85\ dBA$$

Source: The Noise Manual, 5th Edition AIHA

Hearing Conservation

When employees are exposed to noise levels at or above an eight-hour TWA of 85 dBA, or an equivalent dose of 50%, OSHA defines this as the action level for noise. If the action level is reached, enlist all employees who are at or above the action level in a Hearing Conservation Program (HCP).

According to OSHA 1910.95, requirements for a hearing conservation program are:
- Monitoring Program
- Hearing Protection Devices
- Training and Education
- Recordkeeping
- Audiometric Testing

There are three types of threshold shift:
- *Standard Threshold Shift* – A change in hearing threshold relative to the baseline audiogram of 10 dB or more at 2000, 3000 and 4000 Hz in either ear.
- *Temporary Threshold Shift* – A temporary loss in hearing sensitivity as the result of short term exposure to noise or fatigue in the inner ear.
- *Permanent Threshold Shift* – A permanent loss in hearing sensitivity due to the destruction of sensory cells from long term exposure to noise and acoustic trauma.

Sound Intensity Level

$$SPL = 10\,log\left(\frac{I}{I_0}\right)$$

$$L_I = 10log\left(\frac{I}{I_0}\right)$$

Where:

L_I or SPL is the sound pressure level, expressed in dB

I is the sound intensity expressed in $\frac{W}{m^2}$

I_0 is the reference sound intensity expressed in $10^{-12}\,\frac{W}{m^2}$

Use: To find the connection between sound intensity and sound pressure level.

Example:

Calculate the sound pressure level for a measured intensity of 10^{-5} W/m^2 if the reference intensity is 10^{-10} W/m^2.

$$SPL = 10\left(log\frac{I}{I_0}\right)$$

Step 1: Solve for L_i

$$SPL = 10\,log\left(\frac{10^{-5}}{10^{-10}}\right)$$

$$SPL = 50\,dB$$

CIH Exam Study Workbook Volume I

Sound Pressure Level - Sound Power Level Relationship

$$L_P = L_W - 20\log r - 0.5 + DI + CF$$

Where:

L_p is the sound pressure level, expressed as dB

L_W is the power level generated by the source, expressed as dB

r is the distance from the source, expressed as feet

DI is the directivity index

CF is the correction factor to temperature and pressure (assumed to be zero)

Note: CF is shown as T in equations and formula sheet older than 2017

Use: To describe the relationship between the sound pressure level (L_P) and the sound power level (L_W).

Metric: $L_p = L_w - 20\log r - 11 + DI + CF$, with r in meters and other units unchanged.

Example:

In the corner of a large room a machine is generating sound at a power level of 105 dB. Determine the estimated sound pressure level at a distance of 15 feet?

$$L_P = L_W - 20\log r - 0.5 + DI + T$$

$$L_W = 105\ dB$$
$$r = 15\ feet$$
$$DI = 10\log Q$$
$$Q = 8\ (because\ of\ a\ room\ corner)$$
$$T = 0$$
$$DI = 10\log_{10}Q$$

Step 1: Solve for DI

$$DI = 10\log 8$$
$$DI = 9.03$$

Step 2: Solve for L_P

$$L_P = 105 - 20\log 15 - 0.5 + 9.03 + 0$$

$$L_P = 90\ dB$$

Source: Source: Industrial-Occupational Hygiene Calculations: A Professional Reference

Directivity Index (DI)

$$DI = 10\ logQ$$

Where:
DI is the directivity index, expressed as dB
Q is the directivity factor dependent on the configuration of the space in which the source is located

Use: To calculate the sound pressure level (SPL) change for different radiation patterns

Note: Spherical Rotation (Q = 1) free field; ½ Spherical rotation (Q = 2) floor only; ¼ Spherical rotation (Q = 4) floor and wall; 1/8 Spherical rotation (Q = 8) corner and floor

Example:
Determine the directivity index for ¼ spherical rotation?

$$DI = 10\ logQ$$

$$Q = 4$$

Step 1: Solve for DI

$$DI = 10\ log(4)$$

$$DI = 6\ dB$$

Frequency of Noise Produced by Fan

$$f = \frac{(N)(RPM)}{60}$$

Where:

f is the frequency of the fan, expressed as (Hz)
N is the number of blades on the fan
RPM is revolutions per minute for the fan

Use: To determine the frequency of noise produced by a fan, which helps in selection of fans or utilizing controls to reduce noise.

Example:
Calculate the frequency of sound generated by a 12-bladed fan operating at 150 RPM?

$$f = \frac{(N)(RPM)}{60}$$

Step 1: Calculate the Frequency

$$f = 12 \; x \; \frac{150}{60}$$

$$f = 30 \; Hz$$

Frequency of Wavelength

$$f = \frac{c}{\lambda}$$

Where:

f is the frequency of the sound, expressed as (Hz)

c is the speed of sound $\frac{m}{sec}$

λ is the wavelength, which is expressed as meters if the speed of sound is given as meters per second

Use: To calculate the frequency of a wavelength, which aids in control of the sound.

Example:

If the wavelength is 40 cm, what is the frequency of sound in air?

$$f = \frac{c}{\lambda}$$

Step 1: Solve for f

$$f = \frac{344\,\frac{m}{sec}}{0.4m}$$

$$f = 860\ Hz$$

Determining Center Frequencies

$$f_c = \sqrt{f_1 f_2}$$

Where:

f_c is the center frequency of the octave band, expressed as (HZ)
f_1 is the lower frequency of the octave band, expressed as (HZ)
f_2 is the upper frequency of the octave band, expressed as (HZ)

Use: To determine the center frequency of an octave band, which can aid in control selection

Note: The upper band frequency is twice that of the lower band frequency

Example:
Given a lower band frequency of 22.4 Hz and an upper band frequency of 45 Hz, calculate the center frequency of the bandwidth.

$$f_c = \sqrt{f_1 f_2}$$

Step 1: Solve for f_c

$$f_c = \sqrt{22.4 \times 45}$$

$$f_c = 31 \; Hz$$

Upper and Lower Limit

$$f_2 = 2f_1$$

Where:

f_1 is the lower frequency of the octave band, expressed as (HZ)

f_2 is the upper frequency of the octave band, expressed as (HZ)

Use: To calculate the lower or upper band measurement of an octave band.

Example:

If the lower edge of an octave band measurement is 90 Hz, what is the frequency of the upper band-edge?

$$f_2 = 2f_1$$

$$f_1 = 90\ Hz$$

Step 1: Solve for f_2

$$f_2 = 2(90\ Hz)$$

$$f_2 = 180\ Hz$$

Upper, Lower and Center Frequencies

$$f_2 = \sqrt{2}f_1$$

Where:

f_2 is either the center or upper frequency of octave band, expressed as (Hz)
f_1 is either the lower or center frequency of octave band, expressed as (Hz)

Use: To calculate the center of an octave band when the lower or calculate the upper frequency of an octave band when the center frequency is known.

Note: Not on 2017 ABIH formula sheet

Example:

If the lower frequency of an octave band is 50 Hz, what are the center and upper frequencies of this octave band?

$$f_2 = \sqrt{2}f_1$$

Step 1: Calculate the center frequency of the octave band

$$f_2 \text{ is the Center frequency} = \sqrt{2}(50)$$

$$Center\ frequency = 71\ Hz$$

Step 1: Calculate the center frequency of the octave band

$$Upper\ frequency = \sqrt{2}(71)$$

$$Upper\ frequency = 100\ Hz$$

The center frequency equals the square root of 2 x lower frequency, AND
The upper frequency equals the square root of 2 x the center frequency.

Third Octave Band

$$f_2 = \sqrt[3]{2}(f_1)$$

Where:

f_1 is the lower frequency of the 1/3 octave band, expressed as (HZ)

f_2 is the upper frequency of the 1/3 octave band, expressed as (HZ)

Use: To calculate the one-third octave band when octave band analysis does not provide the required level of detail about the noise.

Example:

Calculate the upper edge frequency of a one-third octave band if the lower edge frequency is 71 Hz?

$$f_2 = \sqrt[3]{2}(f_1)$$

Step 1: Solve for f_2

$$f_2 = \sqrt[3]{2}\,(71)$$

$$f_2 = 90\ Hz$$

Rubric 11: Noise Questions

1. What is the frequency of sound generated by a 12-bladed fan operating at 160 RPM?

    A) 32 Hz.
    B) 54 Hz.
    C) 71 kHz.
    D) 9.9 kHz.

2. A company has employees who work 10-hour shifts. What is the ACGIH noise exposure limit for the 10-hour shift?

    A) 80 dBA.
    B) 82 dBA.
    C) 84 dBA.
    D) 86 dBA.

3. An industrial hygienist conducted noise exposure sampling with a sound level meter for an employee during a shift. The test used a 90 dB criterion level with a 5 dB exchange. The noise exposure sampling results are presented in the table below.

Average dBA	90	92	86	84
Exposure Duration (hours)	2	1	3	2

    Calculate the percent dose for the employee during an 8-hour shift.

    A) 70.6
    B) 73.5
    C) 84.0
    D) 91.3

4. A home is located next to a highway that has a sound power of approximately 0.02 Watts. Calculate the sound power level in dB.

    A) 87 dB.
    B) 103 dB.
    C) 110 dB.
    D) 117 dB.

5. Routine exposures to high noise levels in the work place may result in hearing loss. This loss will typically appear first at what frequency on the audiogram?

    A) 250 Hz.
    B) 1000 Hz.
    C) 2000 Hz.
    D) 4000 Hz.

6. If the lower frequency of an octave band is 45 Hz, what are the center and upper frequencies of this octave band?

    A) Center frequency = 71 Hz; Upper frequency= 100 Hz.
    B) Center frequency = 63 Hz; Upper frequency= 90 Hz.
    C) Center frequency = 84 Hz; Upper frequency= 129 Hz.
    D) Center frequency = 90 Hz; Upper frequency= 148 Hz.

7. Company XYZ is planning on adding additional ventilation to an enclosed paint booth. The new ventilation system is composed of two exhaust hoods. These hoods will ensure employees are not overexposed to the hydrocarbons in the paint. The hoods would be situated in the corner of the room and operate at 70 dB. Two other hoods are also in the room and operate at 80 dB. What would the expected noise level be in the paint booth if the new ventilation system is installed?

    A) 70 dB.
    B) 75 dB.
    C) 83 dB.
    D) 92 dB.

8. A worker at a manufacturing company is monitored for noise exposure. The results state that the worker had a dose of 250%. Using the ACGIH criteria, what is the TWA_{eq} exposure in dBA?

    A) 89 dBA.
    B) 94 dBA.
    C) 99 dBA.
    D) 111 dBA.

9. An Industrial Hygienist is conducting a sound level meter survey at an industry. The sound level meter should be set to which weight to assess the noise hazard?

    A) A-weighted.
    B) B-weighted.
    C) C-weighted.
    D) D-weighted.

10. What is considered the maximum peak sound pressure level for employee exposure?

    A) 110 dB.
    B) 120 dB.
    C) 130 dB.
    D) 140 dB.

11. If a noise enclosure is constructed with ¾" plywood, what would be the expected transmission loss at 2000 Hz? Use the Relative Transmission Loss table below.

Approximate Transmission Loss for Materials (dB)

Material	125	250	500	1,000	2,000	4,000
	Hz					
Sheet metal laminate, 2 lb/ft^2, viscoelastic core	15	25	28	32	39	42
Steel, 16 gauge, 2.5 lb/ft^2	21	30	34	37	40	47
Steel, 18 gauge, 2 lb/ft^2	15	19	31	32	35	48
Plywood, ¾ inch, 2 lb/ft^2	24	22	27	28	25	27
Plywood, ¼ inch, 0.7 lb/ft^2	17	15	20	24	28	27
Panels, perforated metal with mineral fiber tile, 4 inch thick	28	34	40	48	56	62
Glass, laminated, ½ inch	23	31	38	40	47	52
Glass, plate. ¼ inch	25	29	33	36	26	35
Fiber tile, filled mineral, $\frac{5}{8}$ inch	30	32	39	43	53	60
Door, hardwood, $2\frac{5}{8}$ inch	26	33	40	43	48	51
Curtains, lead vinyl, 1 ½ lb/ft^2	22	23	25	31	35	42
Concrete block, 6 inch, lightweight, painted	38	36	40	45	50	56
Cinder block, $7\frac{5}{8}$ inch, hollow	33	33	33	39	45	51
Brick, 4 inch	30	36	37	37	37	43

    A) 25 dB.
    B) 10 dB.
    C) 28 dB.
    D) 14 dB.

12. An industrial hygiene technician conducted sampling at a steel mill. The employee has an 8-hour TWA of 98 decibels. The hearing protection the employee was wearing has an NRR of 32 dB. Considering the employee has been trained and is using the hearing protection correctly, what is the employee's estimated noise exposure?

    A) 80 dBA.
    B) 86 dBA.
    C) 91 dBA.
    D) 94 dBA.

13. An employee is exposed to a sound level of 85 dBA. How many hours per day can an employee be exposed to this sound level following OSHA's PEL criteria?

    A) 10
    B) 12
    C) 14
    D) 16

14. There are two common types of sound waves. What are they?

    A) Transverse and Inverse.
    B) Longitudinal and Inverse.
    C) Transverse and Longitudinal.
    D) Longitudinal and Latitudinal.

15. Inner-transduction is a process that changes mechanical waves in a liquid to chemical impulses sent to the brain. What anatomical parts are associated with this process?

    A) Cochlea and Organ of Corti.
    B) Cochlea, Incus and Maleus.
    C) Organ of Corti, Stapes, and Semicircular Canals.
    D) Incus and Stapes.

16. There are several sound level meters (SLMs) utilized in the occupational health and safety field. Which type of SLM is intended for measurements in the field and laboratory, and will have errors not exceeding 1 dB?

    A) Type 0.
    B) Type 1.
    C) Type 2.
    D) Type S.

17. A common type of frequency analysis uses an Octave Band Analyzer (OBA). This type of frequency analysis allows the user to measure frequencies (e.g., is equipped with band-pass filters). The width of the band is called an octave. An octave is where the upper frequency of the band is __________ the lower frequency of the band.

    A) Twice.
    B) Three times.
    C) Five times.
    D) Ten times.

18. A common noise control material is absorbing (e.g., fibrous glass). What type of noise control absorbing material is a very thin piece of material that when hit by sound causes it to vibrate and absorb the sound waves?

    A) Porous.
    B) Diaphragmatic.
    C) Resonant.
    D) Resistant.

19. Select the variable that represents the upper-bound edge of an octave band analysis.

    A) f_2
    B) f_1
    C) f_c
    D) UE

20. Select the preferred method of noise control.

    A) Path interruption.
    B) Reduction at the receiver.
    C) Reduction at the source.
    D) Worker rotation.

Rubric 11: Noise Answers

1. Answer A.
   Explanation:

$$f = \frac{(N)(RPM)}{60}$$

$$N = 12$$
$$RPM = 160$$

Step 1: Calculate the Frequency

$$f = 12 \; x \; \frac{160}{60}$$

$$f = 32 \; Hz$$

Source: Industrial-Occupational Hygiene Calculations: A Professional Reference

2. Answer C.
   Explanation:

$$Time = \frac{8}{2^{\left(\frac{L-85}{3}\right)}}$$

Step 1: Solve for L

$$10 = \frac{8}{2^{\left(\frac{L-85}{3}\right)}}$$

$$2^{\left(\frac{L-85}{3}\right)} = \frac{8}{10}$$

$$log2\left(\frac{L-85}{3}\right) = log\left(\frac{8}{10}\right)$$

$$\left(\frac{L-85}{3}\right)0.30103 = 0.09691$$

$$L = 3\left(\frac{-0.09691}{0.30103}\right) + 85 = 84.0 \; dBA$$

Source: www.OSHA.gov

---

3. Answer B.

    Explanation: The dose is the total time exposed at each noise level divided by the time of exposure allowed at that level.

Average dBA	90	92	86	84
Exposure Duration (hours)	2	1	3	2

Calculate the percent dose for the employee during an 8-hour shift.

Step 1: Calculate T_p for all levels listed in above table

$$T_p = \frac{8}{\left(2^{\left(\frac{L_{AS}-L_C}{ER}\right)}\right)} \; hours$$

$$T_{90} = \frac{8}{\left(2^{\left(\frac{90-90}{5}\right)}\right)} \; hours$$

$$T_{90} = \frac{8}{1}$$

$$T_{90} = 8.0 \; hours$$

$$T_{92} = \frac{8}{\left(2^{\left(\frac{92-90}{5}\right)}\right)} \; hours$$

$$T_{92} = \frac{8}{1.3}$$

$$T_{92} = 6.2 \; hours$$

$$T_{86} = \frac{8}{\left(2^{\left(\frac{86-90}{5}\right)}\right)} \; hours$$

$$T_{86} = \frac{8}{0.57}$$

$$T_{86} = 14 \; hours$$

$$T_{84} = \frac{8}{\left(2^{\left(\frac{84-90}{5}\right)}\right)} \; hours$$

$$T_{84} = \frac{8}{0.44}$$

$$T_{84} = 18.2 \; hours$$

Step 2: Calculate the Percent Dose

$$\%D = 100\left[\frac{C_1}{T_1} + \frac{C_2}{T_2} + \cdots + \frac{C_i}{T_i}\right]$$

$$\%D = 100\left[\frac{2}{8} + \frac{1}{6.2} + \frac{3}{14} + \frac{2}{18.2}\right]$$

$$\%D = 73.5$$

Source: Source: Industrial-Occupational Hygiene Calculations: A Professional Reference

4. Answer B.
Explanation:

$$L_W = 10Log_{10}\frac{W}{W_0}$$

Step 1: Solve for L_W

$$L_W = 10Log_{10}\frac{0.02}{10^{-12}}$$

$$L_W = 103\ dB$$

5. Answer D.
Explanation: The loss associated with occupational noise exposure is called the "4000 Hz" notch. The sensorineural loss appears in the 3000 to 6000 Hz range routinely, but not in all cases.
Source: Gelfand, S. (2001). Auditory System and Related Disorders. Essentials of Audiology (2nd ed.)

6. Answer B.
Explanation:

$$f_2 = \sqrt{2}(f_1)$$

Step 1: Calculate the center frequency of the octave band

$$Center\ frequency = \sqrt{2}(45)$$

$$Center\ frequency = 63\ Hz$$

Step 2: Calculate the upper frequency of the octave band

$$Upper\ frequency = \sqrt{2}(63)$$

$$Upper\ frequency = 90\ Hz$$

Source: Industrial-Occupational Hygiene Calculations: A Professional Reference

---

7. Answer C.
   Explanation:

$$SPL_f = 10 \, log \sum 10^{\frac{SPL}{10}}$$

Step 1: Solve for SPL_f

$$SPL_f = 10 \, log \, 10^{\frac{70}{10}} + 10^{\frac{70}{10}} + 10^{\frac{80}{10}} + 10^{\frac{80}{10}}$$

$$SPL_f = 83 \, dB$$

Source: Occupational Safety Calculations: A Professional Reference, 2nd Edition

8. Answer A.
   Explanation:

$$TWA_{eq} = 10 \, log \left(\frac{D\%}{100}\right) + 85$$

Step 1: Solve for TWA_{eq}

$$TWA_{eq} = 10 \, log \left(\frac{250}{100}\right) + 85$$

$$TWA_{eq} = 10 \, log(2.5) + 85$$

$$TWA_{eq} = 10(0.40) + 85$$
$$TWA_{eq} = 89 \, dBA$$

Source: Occupational Safety Calculations: A Professional Reference, 2nd Edition

9. Answer A.
   Explanation: The A-weighted sound level measurement has become popular in the assessment of overall noise hazard because it provides a rating of industrial broadband noises that indicates the injurious effects such noise has on human hearing.

   The A-weighted sound level has been adopted as the measurement for assessing noise exposure by the American Conference of Governmental Industrial Hygienists (ACGIH). The A-weighted sound level as the preferred unit of measurement was also adopted by the U.S. Department of Labor as part of its Occupational Safety and Health Standards. The A-weighted sound level has also been shown to provide reasonably good assessments of speech interference and community disturbance conditions and has been adopted by the U.S. Environmental Protection Agency (EPA) for these purposes.
   Source: Fundamentals of Industrial Hygiene

10. Answer D.

Explanation: Impact-type noise is a sharp burst of sound, and sophisticated instrumentation is necessary to determine the peak levels for this type of noise. Noise types other than steady ones are commonly encountered. In general, sounds repeated more than once per second can be considered as steady. Impulsive or impact noise, such as that made by hammer blows or explosions, is generally less than one-half second in duration and does not repeat more often than once per second. Employees should not be exposed to impulsive or impact noise that exceeds a peak sound pressure level of 140 dB.
Source: Fundamentals of Industrial Hygiene

11. Answer D.

Table: Approximate Transmission Loss for Materials (dB)

Material	125	250	500	1,000	2,000	4,000
				Hz		
Sheet metal laminate, 2 lb/ft^2, viscoelastic core	15	25	28	32	39	42
Steel, 16 gauge, 2.5 lb/ft^2	21	30	34	37	40	47
Steel, 18 gauge, 2 lb/ft^2	15	19	31	32	35	48
Plywood, ¾ inch, 2 lb/ft^2	24	22	27	28	25	27
Plywood, ¼ inch, 0.7 lb/ft^2	17	15	20	24	28	27
Panels, perforated metal with mineral fiber tile, 4 inch thick	28	34	40	48	56	62
Glass, laminated, ½ inch	23	31	38	40	47	52
Glass, plate. ¼ inch	25	29	33	36	26	35
Fiber tile, filled mineral, $\frac{5}{8}$ inch	30	32	39	43	53	60
Door, hardwood, $2\frac{5}{8}$ inch	26	33	40	43	48	51
Curtains, lead vinyl, 1 ½ lb/ft^2	22	23	25	31	35	42
Concrete block, 6 inch, lightweight, painted	38	36	40	45	50	56
Cinder block, $7\frac{5}{8}$ inch, hollow	33	33	33	39	45	51
Brick, 4 inch	30	36	37	37	37	43

Explanation:

Step 1: Locate the value on the table for the ¾ inch plywood row and 2000 Hz column: 25 dB

Step 2: Solve for TL

$$TL = 10 \, log\left(\frac{1}{\tau}\right)$$

$$TL = 10 \, log\left(\frac{1}{25}\right)$$

$$TL = -14 \, dB$$

The question asks for the transmission loss, so 14 dB is correct.

12. Answer B.

Explanation: Noise Reduction Ratings are found in the OSHA Technical Manual. When OSHA promulgated its Hearing Conservation Amendment in 1983, it incorporated the EPA labeling requirements for hearing protectors (40 CFR 211), which required manufacturers to identify the noise reduction capability of all hearing protectors on the hearing protector package. This measure is referred to as the noise reduction rating (NRR). It is a laboratory derived numerical estimate of the attenuation achieved by the protector. It became apparent that the amount of actual protection in the workplace with the designated hearing protectors did not correlate with the attenuation indicated by the NRR. OSHA acknowledged that in most cases, this number overstated the protection afforded to workers and required the application for certain circumstances of a safety factor of 50% to the NRR, above and beyond the 7 dB subtraction called for when using A-weighted measurements.

For example, consider a worker who is exposed to 98 dBA for 8 hours and whose hearing protectors have an NRR of 25 dB. We can estimate the worker's resultant exposure using the 50% safety factor. The worker's resultant exposure is 89 dBA in this case.

The 50% safety factor adjusts labeled NRR values for workplace conditions and is used when considering whether engineering controls are to be implemented.

$$Estimated\ dBA\ exposure = TWA(dBA) - [(25 - 7)\ x\ 50\%] = 89\ dBA$$

Though using the 50% safety factor produces the most reliable result, it is not used for enforcement purposes. For enforcement purposes, CSHOs should subtract 7 dB from the NRR without considering the 50% safety factor.

Rewriting the above formula to divide by 2 rather than multiply by 50%:

$$Estimated\ Noise\ Exposure = TWA - \left(\frac{NRR - 7}{2}\right)$$

Step 1: Solve for Estimated Noise Exposure

$$Estimated\ Noise\ Exposure = 98 - \left(\frac{32 - 7}{2}\right)$$

$$Estimated\ Noise\ Exposure = 98 - 12.5$$

$$Estimated\ Noise\ Exposure = 86\ dBA$$

Source: OSHA Technical Manual

13. Answer D.

Explanation:

Allowable noise exposure

OSHA 5 decibel (dBb) Exchange	ACGIH 3 decibel (db) Exchange
105 db → 1 hour	94 db → 1 hour
100 db → 2 hours	91 db → 2 hours
95 db → 4 hours	88 db → 4 hours
90 db → 8 hours	85 db → 8 hours
85 db → 16 hours	82 db → 16 hours

Note: Neither incorporate sounds levels under 80 db into dose.

14. Answer C.

Explanation: The two common types of sound waves are transverse waves and longitudinal waves. Transverse waves move horizontally and molecules move vertically. Longitudinal waves move vertically and molecules move horizontally. Sound waves are created by vibration. You can change their amplitude and frequency, but you cannot change the speed at which they travel through a medium. They are a constant that varies with temperature (i.e., the speed of sound for a given medium and temperature is constant).
Source: Industrial Hygiene Reference and Study Guide, 3ʳᵈ edition

15. Answer A.

Explanation: The two anatomical parts associated with the inner-transduction process are the cochlea and the organ of corti. The cochlea transforms the sound into a neural message. The function of the cochlea is to transform the vibrations of the cochlear liquids and associated structures into a neural signal. The organ of corti is the essential receptor end organ for hearing (contains the hair cells).
Source: Industrial Hygiene Reference and Study Guide, 3ʳᵈ edition

16. Answer B.

Explanation: *Type 0 (Laboratory standard)*: Intended for use in the laboratory as a high-precision reference standard and is not required to satisfy environmental requirements for a field instrument. *Type 1 (Precision)*: Intended for measurements in the field and in the laboratory. Should have errors not exceeding 1 dB. *Type 2 (General purpose)*: A more lenient tolerance than Type 1 and intended for general field use, particularly in applications where high-frequency (over 10 kHz) sound components are not predominant. Estimated errors will not exceed 2 dB. *Type S (Special purpose)*: May have design tolerances associated with any of the three grades but is not required to contain all of the functions stipulated for a numbered type.
Sources: Earshen, J.J. "Sound Measurement: Instrumentation and Noise Descriptors." The Noise Manual, 5ᵗʰ Edition.

17. Answer A.

    Explanation: The width of the band is called an octave. An octave is where the upper frequency of the band is twice the lower frequency of the band.
    Source: Industrial Hygiene Reference and Study Guide, 3rd edition

18. Answer B.

    Explanation: There are three different types of noise absorbing control materials: porous, diaphragmatic, and resonant. Porous absorbing noise control material allows acoustic energy to enter the pores to cause fibers to move and change the energy to heat. It is good for high-frequency noise. Diaphragmatic absorbing noise control materials are thin materials that vibrate and absorb the sound waves and are is good for controlling low-frequency noise. Resonant absorbing noise control material utilize air pockets that convert sound waves into heat.
    Source: Industrial Hygiene Reference and Study Guide, 3rd edition

19. Answer A.

    Explanation:

    $f_c = \sqrt{(f_1 f_2)}$ where f_c is the center frequency, f_1 is the edge of the lower frequency, and f_2 is the upper band edge frequency.
    Source: Noise and Hearing Conservation Manual, 4th Edition

20. Answer C.

    Explanation: By controlling at the source, the use of hearing protection devices may be eliminated. If effective, audiometric testing and other actions may be reduced.
    Source: Noise and Hearing Conservation Manual, 4th Edition

Rubric 12: Non-Engineering Controls

In occupational health and safety, the hierarchy of controls is important for guiding professionals in the selection of hazard control methods. Historically, the hierarchy was engineered controls, administrative controls, and personal protective equipment. More recently, ANSI Z-10 lists the hierarchy of controls as elimination, substitution, engineering controls, administrative controls and personal protective equipment.

Elimination of the hazard during the planning and design phase is considered the optimal choice, with substitution of less hazardous materials and machinery being desirable as well. When hazardous agents cannot be removed, then engineered controls including ventilation, containment, and other methods must be utilized. When these efforts are not effective at reducing the hazard to acceptable levels, the non-engineered controls are used.

Non-engineered controls include administrative controls and personal protective equipment. Administrative controls include training, education, warnings, scheduling and other hazard management techniques. Personal protective equipment includes materials and devices that are worn or used by the worker to reduce the hazard to the worker. Personal protective equipment use has several limitations, including potential discomfort, physiological strain, user diligence, and in the event of failure, exposure occurs.

The majority of the injuries and exposures related to dermal hazards can be controlled by the appropriate selection and use of protective clothing (and additional control measures). Protective clothing is utilized in various combinations. Commonly used protective clothing includes gloves, boots, and garments. Failure to identify the appropriate equipment and verify the proper use can result in harm. Protective clothing can be to protect the worker from thermal, fire, abrasion, cuts, vibration, chemical, biological and radiological hazards.

When engineered and administrative controls fail to reduce the risk of inhalation hazards to an acceptable level respiratory protection must be used. To function as intended, respirators must be properly selected, fit-tested, maintained, and used by trained employees. A respiratory protection program should be established and implemented based on the performance limitations and capabilities of the respirators, as well as regulations and standards.

Important Terms and Concepts

Administrative controls- Methods of controlling employee exposures by job rotation, work assignment, time periods away from the hazard, or training in specific work practices designed to reduce the exposure.

Assigned Protection Factor (APF) - The expected workplace level of respiratory protection that would be provided by a properly functioning respirator or a class of respirators to properly fitted and trained users.

Assigned Protection Factors					
Type of Respirator	**Quarter mask**	**Half mask**	**Full facepiece**	**Helmet/Hood**	**Loose-fitting facepiece**
1. *Air-Purifying Respirator*	5	10	50	—	—
2. *Powered Air-Purifying Respirator (PAPR)*	—	50	1,000	25/1,000	25
3. *Supplied-Air Respirator (SAR) or Airline Respirator*					
• Demand mode	—	10	50	— 25/1,000	— 25
• Continuous flow mode	—	50	1,000	—	—
• Pressure-demand or other positive-pressure mode	—	50	1,000		
4. *Self-Contained Breathing Apparatus (SCBA)*					
• Demand mode	—	10	50	50	—
• Pressure-demand or other positive- pressure mode (e.g., open/closed circuit)	—	—	10,000	10,000	—

Recreated from OSHA 3352-02 2009 Assigned Protection Factors for the Revised Respiratory Protection Standard.

Breakthrough time- The time elapsed from the initial contact of the chemical on the outside surface until detection on the inside surface.

Chemical cartridge- The type of absorption unit used with a respirator for removal of low concentrations of specific vapors and gases.

Degradation- A deleterious change in one or more physical properties of a protective material caused by contact with a chemical.

Hazard- A condition, set of circumstances, or inherent property that can cause injury, illness, or death.

High-efficiency particulate air filter (HEPA)- One that is at least 99.97 percent efficient in removing thermally generated monodisperse dioctyl phthalate smoke particles with a diameter of 0.0003 mm.

Incident- An event in which a work-related injury or illness (regardless of severity) or fatality occurred or could have occurred (commonly referred to as a "close call" or "near miss").

Fit factor- A quantitative measure of the fit of a particular respirator to a particular individual.

Fit test- The use of a challenge agent to evaluate the fit of a respirator on an individual.

Immediately dangerous to life or health (IDLH) - Any atmosphere that poses an immediate hazard to life or poses immediate, irreversible, and debilitating effects on health.

Lockout/tagout- A basic safety concept and OSHA standard requiring implementation of practices and procedures to prevent the release of potentially hazardous energy from machines or parts of machines and equipment while maintenance, servicing, or alteration activity is performed. The energy in question may be electrical, mechanical, chemical, or any other form.

Maximum use concentration (MUC) - Chemical cartridges and canisters are limited to use in concentrations that are no greater than the assigned protection factor of the respirator times the occupational exposure limit.

Penetration – The flow of chemicals through zippers, seams, or holes in the protective clothing at the non-molecular level.

Personal protective equipment- Devices worn by the worker to protect against hazards in the environment (e.g., respirators, gloves, and hearing protectors).

Permeation – The movement of a chemical through a protective clothing item that does not have any visible holes.

Permeation Rate – The rate of movement of a chemical through the barrier stated as mass/area/time, such as µg/cm/minute. ASTM publishes a method for testing the permeation of protective clothing (F739-07).

Preventive action- Action taken to reduce the likelihood that an underlying system deficiency or hazard will occur or recur in another similar process. (Fix a potential problem.)

Risk- An estimate of the combination of the likelihood of an occurrence of a hazardous event or exposure(s), and the severity of injury or illness that may be caused by the event or exposure.

Qualitative fit-test- A pass/fail fit-test that relies on the subject's sensory response to detect the challenge agent.

Quantitative fit-test- A fit-test that uses an instrument to measure the challenge agent inside and outside the respirator.

Respirator- A device to protect the wearer from inhalation of harmful contaminants. Interposed material (such as a wall) that protects workers from harmful radiations released by radioactive materials.

Rubric 12: Non-Engineering Controls Questions

1. Workers must use respiratory protection due to the presence of harmful vapors in air despite the implementation of engineered controls that include ventilation. The elastomeric ½ face respirator used for the previous three years has been discontinued by the manufacturer. After reviewing the available respirators, a different elastomeric ½ face respirator is selected. Best practice dictates that the following should be performed prior to issuing the new respirator to the workers.

    A) Collect the old respirators for redistribution.
    B) Fit-test the workers for the new respirator.
    C) Fit-test and train the workers for the new respirator.
    D) Fit-test, train and photograph the workers while wearing the new respirator.

2. Some of the requirements of ANSI Z87.1 are testing, normal, high-velocity & mass impact, penetration, flammability resistance, ease of cleaning, and minimum thickness. The ANSI document is related to:

    A) Foot protection.
    B) Hearing protection.
    C) Head protection.
    D) Eye and face protection.

3. ANSI Z 89.1 addresses protective headwear for industrial workers. The headwear is tested for penetration resistance, flammability and ________________.

    A) Chemical resistance.
    B) Radiant heat transfer.
    C) Electrical hazards.
    D) Resistance to UV degradation.

4. Fault Tree Analysis involves deductive rather than inductive reasoning. Select the best description of the process.

    A) Cost effective use of teams and design information.
    B) A fire and explosion index.
    C) A generic approach to quantitative risk and hazard analysis methods.
    D) Starts with the outcome event and works backwards to find the initiating event or events.

5. Choose the type of control that is the first choice in mitigating employee exposure to occupational hazards.

    A) Personal protective equipment.
    B) Administrative controls.
    C) Eliminate the hazard.
    D) Substitute for less-hazardous substances.

---

6. The type of equipment that provides the best foot protection from falling objects is:

    A) Phalange protection.
    B) Metatarsal protection.
    C) Boot standards following ANSI Z89.1.
    D) Steel toe boots.

7. Which respirator has the highest assigned protection factor?

    A) Air-purifying respirator (APR)- half mask.
    B) Air-purifying respirator (APR)- full facepiece.
    C) Powered air-purifying respirator (PAPR)- half mask.
    D) Powered air-purifying respirator (PAPR)- full facepiece.

8. What is the required optical density to lower laser irradiance by a factor of 10,000?

    A) 1.0
    B) 2.0
    C) 3.0
    D) 4.0

9. Choose the class of hard hat that should be used to provide protection from falling objects and electrical shock from low voltages.

    A) Class A.
    B) Class C.
    C) Class E.
    D) Class G.

10. ANSI Z88.2-1992 assigned a protection factor of _____ for a demand full-face self-contained breathing apparatus (SCBA). NOTE: Z88.2 was revised in 2015 and the assigned protection factors are aligned with OSHA in the revision.

    A) 10
    B) 100
    C) 1,000
    D) 10,000

11. Fit testing should be performed for:

    A) Positive pressure respirators only.
    B) Negative pressure respirators only.
    C) All tight-fitting respirators.
    D) All respirators.

12. __________ is described as the diffusion of chemicals through intact chemical protective clothing.

 A) Degradation.
 B) Penetration.
 C) Permeation.
 D) Infiltration.

13. The Occupational Safety and Health Administration (OSHA) defines an IDLH value in their hazardous waste operations and emergency response regulation as follows:

An atmospheric concentration of any toxic, corrosive or asphyxiant substance that poses an immediate threat to life or would cause irreversible or delayed adverse health effects or would interfere with an individual's ability to escape from a dangerous atmosphere. [29 CFR 1910.120]

In the OSHA regulation on permit-required confined spaces, an IDLH condition is defined as follows:

Any condition that poses an immediate or delayed threat to life or that would cause irreversible adverse health effects or that would interfere with an individual's ability to escape unaided from a permit space. **Note**: *Some materials--hydrogen fluoride gas and cadmium vapor, for example--may produce immediate transient effects that, even if severe, may pass without medical attention, but are followed by sudden, possibly fatal collapse 12-72 hours after exposure. The victim "feels normal" from recovery from transient effects until collapse. Such materials in hazardous quantities are considered to be "immediately dangerous to life or health."*

ANSI considers confined space IDLH if the oxygen concentration is less than:

 A) 10.5%
 B) 15.8%
 C) 19.5%
 D) 20.9%

14. Airlines shall not exceed the length of _______ when supplying air to type C respirators.

 A) 100 feet.
 B) 200 feet.
 C) 300 feet.
 D) 400 feet.

15. The partial pressure of oxygen in a normal atmosphere at sea level is:

    A) 142 mm Hg.
    B) 160 mm Hg.
    C) 189 mm Hg.
    D) 193 mm Hg.

16. Which of the following would not be considered an acceptable administrative control for worker exposures to chemicals?

    A) Employee training.
    B) Worker rotation.
    C) Reduced work times.
    D) All are acceptable.

17. What factor listed below is the least likely to affect the cartridge life of respirator chemical cartridges?

    A) Relative humidity.
    B) Work rate.
    C) Workplace temperature.
    D) Chemical concentration.

18. In the absence of manufacturer documentation that the assigned protection factor is 1000, what is the assigned protection factor for a helmet-type powered air purifying respirator equipped with a face-piece shroud?

    A) 5
    B) 10
    C) 20
    D) 25

19. Select the statement that best describes the maximum use concentration.

    A) The maximum atmospheric concentration of a hazardous substance from which an employee can be expected to be protected when wearing a respirator.
    B) The maximum amount of air an employee can inhale of a hazardous substance without demonstrating adverse health effects.
    C) The maximum amount of time an employee has before demonstrating adverse health effects.
    D) The maximum atmospheric concentration of a hazardous substance from which an employee can be expected to not be protected when wearing a respirator.

20. Which statement is false in regard to quantitative fit testing?

    A) Measures fit factors greater than 10,000.
    B) Requires a probed face piece or probe adaptor.
    C) The fit test subject can provide a false response to the test.
    D) Fits any tight-fitting respirator.

Rubric 12: Non-Engineering Controls Answers

1. Answer C.
   Explanation: Fit-test and training are critical requirements. A photograph is not of significant value. The workers must also demonstrate the ability to properly use the new respirator.
   Industrial Hygiene Reference and Study Guide, 3rd edition

2. Answer D.
   Explanation: Z87.1 – 1989: American National Standard Practice for Occupational and Educational Eye and Face Protection.
   Industrial Hygiene Reference and Study Guide, 3rd edition

3. Answer C.
   Explanation: Head protection consists of two types: **Type I and Type II**

   Type I hard hats are only designed to protect workers from objects and blows that come from above and strike the top of a helmet.

   Type II hard hats are designed to offer protection from lateral blows and objects. This includes from the front, back, and side as well as from the top. Type II hard hats are also tested for off-center penetration resistance and chin strap retention.

   Classes
   Hard hats are also divided into classes that indicate how well they protect against electrical shock.
   - Class E (Electrical) hard hats can withstand up to 20,000 volts of electricity
   - Class G (General) hard hats are able to withstand 2,200 volts of electricity
   - Class C (Conductive) hard hats offer no protection from electric shock

   There were three main changes to the ANSI/ISEA Z89.1-2014 standard issued on May 15, 2014:

   - Under the section of *Accessories and Replacement Components,* there is further clarification that accessory or component manufacturers are required to prove that their components do not cause the helmets to fail. Helmet accessory or component suppliers must provide justification upon request that their product would not cause the helmet to fail the requirements of the Head Protection Standard.

   - Some additional language added under the *Instructions* and *Markings* section to help clarify that "useful service life" for helmets is not required by the Standard. It is up to helmet manufacturers if they want to include specific service life in terms of years. Manufacturers could elect to specify the number of years for their helmet's service life or elect to identify certain conditions that may affect a helmet's protection capability over time.

          Copyright©2019 SPAN International Training, LLC

- The last section revised was the Higher Temperature section for users who work in hot environments. This section was updated to incorporate an optional preconditioning at a higher temperature of 140° F +/- 3.6° F (60° C +/- 2° C). Previously hot temperature preconditioning was conducted at 120° F +/- 3.6° F (48.8° C +/- 2° C) under the 2009 Standard. Helmets that meet the performance criteria after being preconditioned to these higher temperatures (140° F) will be designated with a HT marking.

4. Answer D.
   Explanation: HAZOPS can be cost effective for complex hazards and use of teams and design information. Dow and MOND are fire and explosion indices. HAZAN is a generic TERM for various quantitative risk and hazard analysis methods. Fault tree starts with the outcome event and works backwards to find the initiating event or events. It uses Boolean logic.
   Source: The Occupational Environment: Its Evaluation, Control and Management, 3rd edition

5. Answer C.
   Explanation: Controlling exposures to occupational hazards is the fundamental method of protecting workers. Hierarchy of controls is utilized to determine how to implement feasible and effective control solutions. The hierarchy of controls include the following: 1) eliminate the hazard 2) substitute with less-hazardous substances 3) engineered controls 4) administrative controls, and 5) personal protective equipment.
   Source: ANSI Z10 and CDC/NIOSH

6. Answer B.
   Explanation: Steel toe boots provide some protection, but do not protect the entire foot. Boots with metatarsal protection have a protective plate covering the foot and ankle. (Note: ANSIZ89.1 is the standard for hard hats.)
   Source: OSHA Personal Protective Equipment

7. Answer D.
   Explanation: Assigned protection factors are set in OSHA's respiratory protection standard 29 CFR 1910.134. See the table below for the assigned protection factors for each type of respirator.

Type of Respirator	Half Mask	Full Face Piece
Air-purifying respirator (APR)	10	50
Powered air-purifying respirator (PAPR)	50	1,000

   Source: CFR 1910.134; osha.gov

8. Answer B.
   Explanation:

$$OD = log\left(\frac{I_o}{I}\right)$$

$$\frac{I_o}{I} = 10,000$$

Step 1: Solve for Optical Density

$$OD = log(10,000)$$
$$OD = 4.0$$

9. Answer D.
   Explanation: ANSI Z89.1-2009 has the following hard hat classifications.
   - Class G hard hats are for electrical use with low voltages (2,200 volts).
   - Class E hard hats can be used with high voltages (22,000 volts).
   - Class C hard hats conduct electricity and provide no electrical protection.
   Source: American National Standards Institute (ANSI) Z89.12009

10. Answer B.
    Explanation:

Table: Assigned Protection Factors ANSI Z88.2-1992

Type of Respirator	Half Mask	Full Face piece
Air Purifying	10	100
Atmosphere Supplying- SCBA (Demand)	10	100
Atmosphere Supplying- Airline (Demand)	10	100

Source: ANSI Z88.2-1992

11. Answer C.
    Explanation: 1910.134(f)(1): The employer should ensure that employees using a tight-fitting face piece respirator are fit tested prior to initial use of the respirator, whenever a different respirator face piece (size, style, model or make) is used, and at least annually thereafter.
    Source: osha.gov

12. Answer C.
    Explanation: Permeation is the process by which a contaminant migrates through a protective clothing material on a molecular level.
    Source: Fundamentals of Industrial Hygiene, 5th Edition

13. Answer D.

    Explanation: ANSI Z88.27.3.3- Special considerations for confined spaces. Confined spaces continue to be the cause of numerous deaths and serious injuries. Therefore, any confined space containing less than 20.9% oxygen is to be considered IDLH, unless the source of the oxygen reduction is understood and controlled.
    Source: OSHA.gov &American National Standards Institute

14. Answer C.

    Explanation: Type C airline respirators are supplied with breathing air from a compressor or a large cylinder that provides air at a maximum of 125 psi using a maximum of 300 feet of hose.
    Source: osha.gov

15. Answer B.

    Explanation: Inspired air is 21% oxygen. Atmospheric pressure at sea level is 760 mm Hg. Therefore, the partial pressure of oxygen in a normal atmosphere at sea level is 160 mm Hg.

$$.21 \ x \ 760 \ mm \ Hg \ = \ 160 \ mm \ Hg$$

16. Answer D.

    Explanation: Administrative controls that reduce employee exposures by scheduling reduced work times and worker rotation in contaminant areas. Employee training that includes hazard recognition and specific work practices that help reduce exposure is also valid.
    Source: Fundamentals of Industrial Hygiene, 2nd Edition

17. Answer C.

    Explanation: Workplace temperature is the least likely to affect cartridge life of respirator chemical cartridges. All of the above have an effect on the service life of a cartridge, with relative humidity having a major effect. A safety factor of 2 is recommended for RH above 65%, and experimental testing is recommended at levels at 85% or more. Increased temperature without an increase in RH may loosen attractive forces for the media to the contaminant. Another important factor is the volume of activated carbon in the cartridge.
    Source: OHSA.gov/SLTC/respiratory

18. Answer D.

Explanation: See the OSHA APF and the answer is 25, but ANSI Z88.2-1992 provides a different factor based on filter used. None of the ANSI APFs are choices in the question.

Assigned Protection Factors					
Type of Respirator	**Quarter mask**	**Half mask**	**Full facepiece**	**Helmet/Hood**	**Loose-fitting facepiece**
1. *Air-Purifying Respirator*	5	10	50	—	—
2. *Powered Air-Purifying Respirator (PAPR)*	—	50	1,000	25/1,000	25
3. *Supplied-Air Respirator (SAR) or Airline Respirator*					
• Demand mode	—	10	50	— 25/1,000	— 25
• Continuous flow mode	—	50	1,000	—	—
• Pressure-demand or other positive-pressure mode	—	50	1,000		
4. *Self-Contained Breathing Apparatus (SCBA)*					
• Demand mode	—	10	50	50	—
• Pressure-demand or other positive- pressure mode (e.g., open/closed circuit	—	—	10,000	10,000	—

Recreated from OSHA 3352-02 2009 Assigned Protection Factors for the Revised Respiratory Protection Standard.

19. Answer A.

Explanation: 1910.134: Maximum use concentration (MUC) means the maximum atmospheric concentration of a hazardous substance from which an employee can be expected to be protected when wearing a respirator; it is determined by the assigned protection factor of the respirator or class of respirators and the exposure limit of the hazardous substance. The MUC can be determined mathematically by multiplying the assigned protection factor specified for a respirator by the required OSHA permissible exposure limit, short-term exposure limit, or ceiling limit. When no OSHA exposure limit is available for a hazardous substance, an employer must determine an MUC on the basis of relevant available information and informed professional judgment.

Source: osha.gov

        Copyright©2019 SPAN International Training, LLC

20. Answer C.

   Explanation: Portacount fit testing is utilized for quantitative fit testing, and it is possible to measure a fit factor greater than 10,000.

   Advantages of quantitative fit testing: No protection-factor limit, documentation of numerical results, eliminates chance of employee deception or bluffing.

   Disadvantages of quantitative fit testing: Expensive up-front equipment costs, requires probed face piece or probe adapter, and annual recalibration of equipment is suggested.

   OSHA recognizes three types of quantitative fit testing protocol agents: generated aerosol, ambient aerosol condensation nuclei count (CNC), and controlled negative pressure (CNP). All three types of quantitative fit testing use a digital instrument that measures airborne particles inside and outside the test respirator, or measures vacuum pressure. A special sampling probe takes measurements inside the mask.
   Source: tsi.com and OSHA.gov

Reference List

Anna, Daniel H. The Occupational Environment: Its Evaluation, Control and Management. Fairfax, VA: American Industrial Hygiene Association, 2011. Print.

ANSI/ ASSE Z10 (2012). American National Standard for Occupational Health & Safety Management Systems. Des Plaines, Illinois: American Society of Safety Engineers. Print.

Bingham, Eula, Barbara Cohrssen, and F. A. Patty. Patty's Toxicology. Hoboken, NJ: Wiley, A John Wiley & Sons, 2012. Print.

Brown, Theodore L., Bruce Edward. Bursten, and LeMay, Harold. Chemistry: The Central Science. Upper Saddle River: Prentice-Hall International, 2000. Print.

Burton, D. J. Industrial Hygiene Workbook: The Occupational Health Sciences. Bountiful, UT: Carr Printing, 2003. Print.

ABIH. American Board of Industrial Hygiene. Web.

ACGIH Industrial Ventilation Handbook, Manual of Recommended Practices, American Conference of Governmental Industrial Hygienists.

ACGIH, Threshold Limit Values and Biological Exposure Indices.

Engelhardt, Susan J., Judith M. Grunewald, Ralph Grunewald, Dee A. Kaiser, and Joshua P. Walkowicz. Radiation Protection, A Practical Guide. Print.

EPA. United States Environmental Protection Agency. Web.

Fleeger, Allan K., and Dean R. Lillquist. Industrial Hygiene Reference & Study Guide. Fairfax, VA: American Industrial Hygiene Association, 2011. Print.

Hathaway, Gloria J., Nick H. Proctor, James P. Hughes, and Michael L. Fischman. Proctor and Hughes' Chemical Hazards of the Workplace. 3rd ed. Print.

Jahn, Steven D., William H. Bullock, and Joselito S. Ignacio. A Strategy for Assessing and Managing Occupational Exposures. Fairfax, VA: AIHA, 2015. Print.

Klaassen, Curtis D., Toxicology, The Basic Science of Poisons, Casarett and Doull's, 7th ed. Print.

NIOSH. The National Institute for Occupational Safety and Health. Centers for Disease Control and Prevention. Centers for Disease Control and Prevention. Web.

OSHA. Occupational Safety and Health Administration. United States Department of Labor. Web.

Pagano, Marcello. Principles of Biostatistics. 2nd ed. Pacific Grove: Brooks/Cole, 2012. Print.

Plog, Barbara A., and Patricia Quinlan. Fundamentals of Industrial Hygiene. Itasca: National Safety Council, 2012. Print.

Stern, M.B, and S.Z Mansdorf. Applications and Computational Elements of Industrial Hygiene. Boca Raton,FL: Lewis, 1999. Print.

Stewart, James et al, Industrial Hygiene Calculations: A Professional Reference. Millennium Publishing. Print.